Table of Contents

Digestive System of Cat

Bones of The Cat

Skeletal System of Cat

Respiratory System of Cat

Internal Organs of Cat

Heart & Blood Vessels of Cat

Lymphatic System of Cat

Nervous System of Cat

Reproductive Systems of Cat

Endocrine System of Cat

Urogenital System of Cat

Organ System of Cat

Endocrine Glands of Cat

Brain Anatomy of Cat

Skull Anatomy of Cat

Heart Anatomy of Cat

Lung Anatomy of Cat

Ear Anatomy of Cat

Eye Anatomy of Cat

Cross-Section of Eye

Cat Hind Leg Bone

Cat Nail Anatomy

How To Trim Cat's Nails

Gonads & Genital Tract of Cat

Skeleton Anatomy of Cat

Venous System of Cat

And Many More....

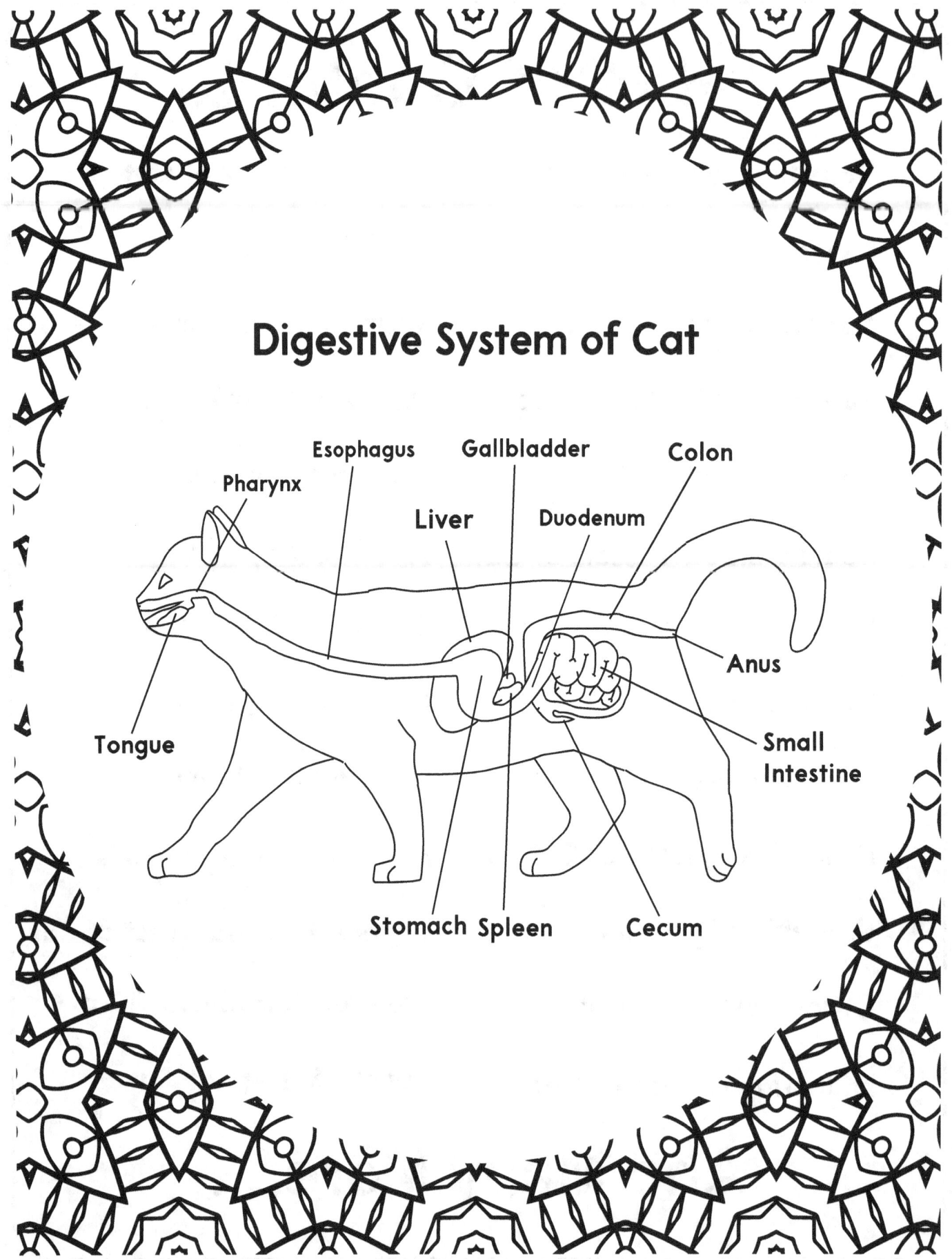

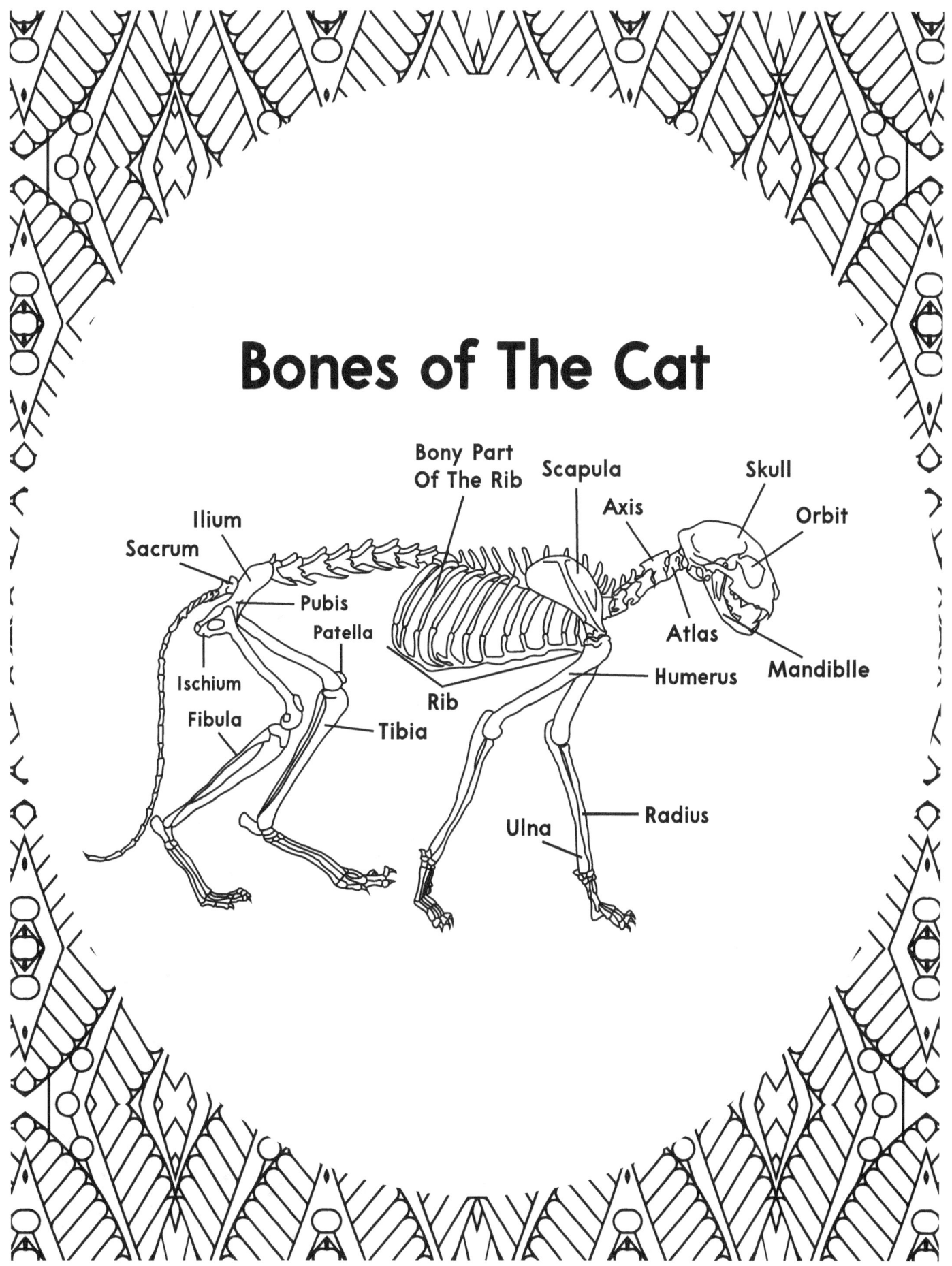

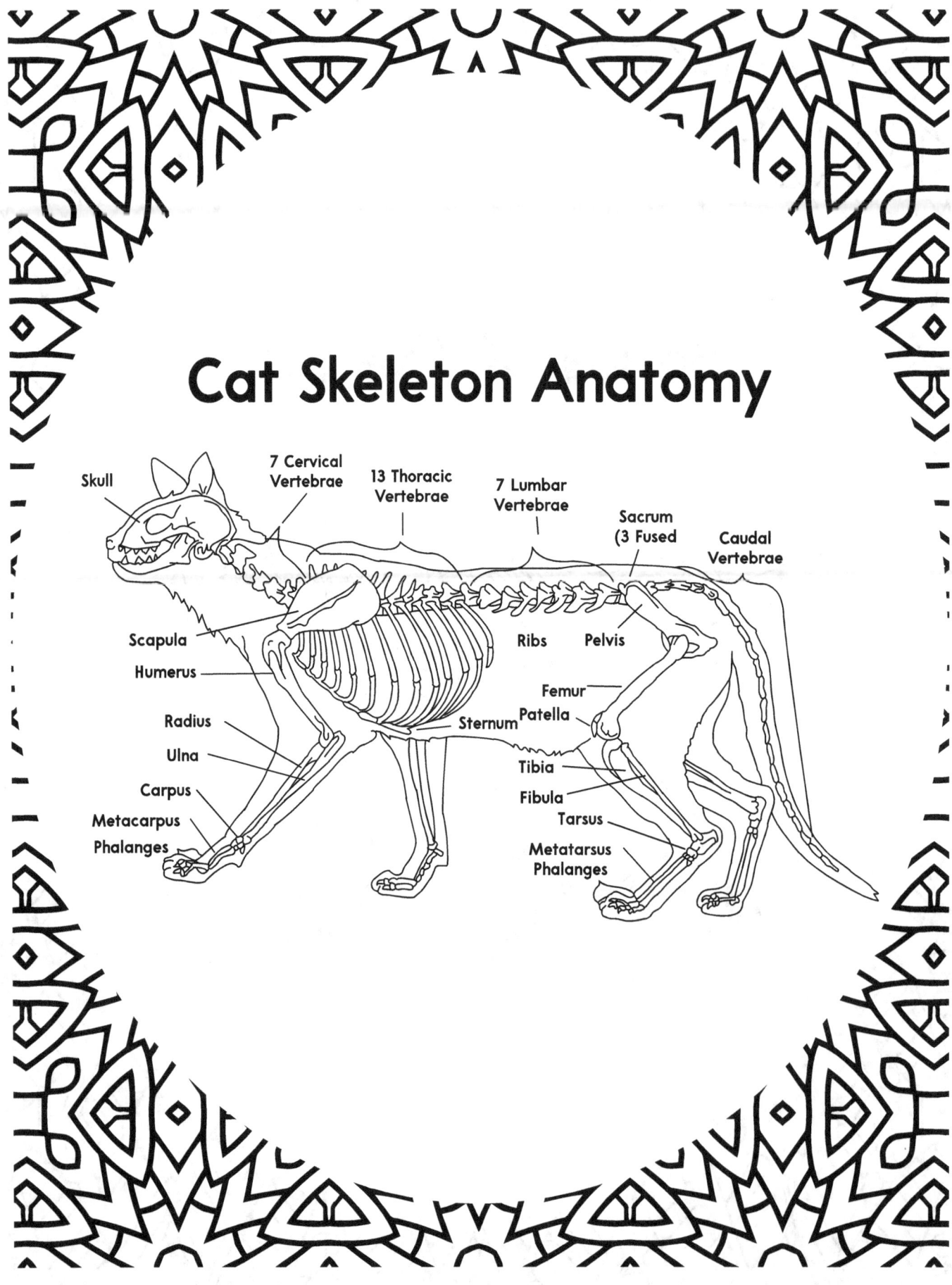

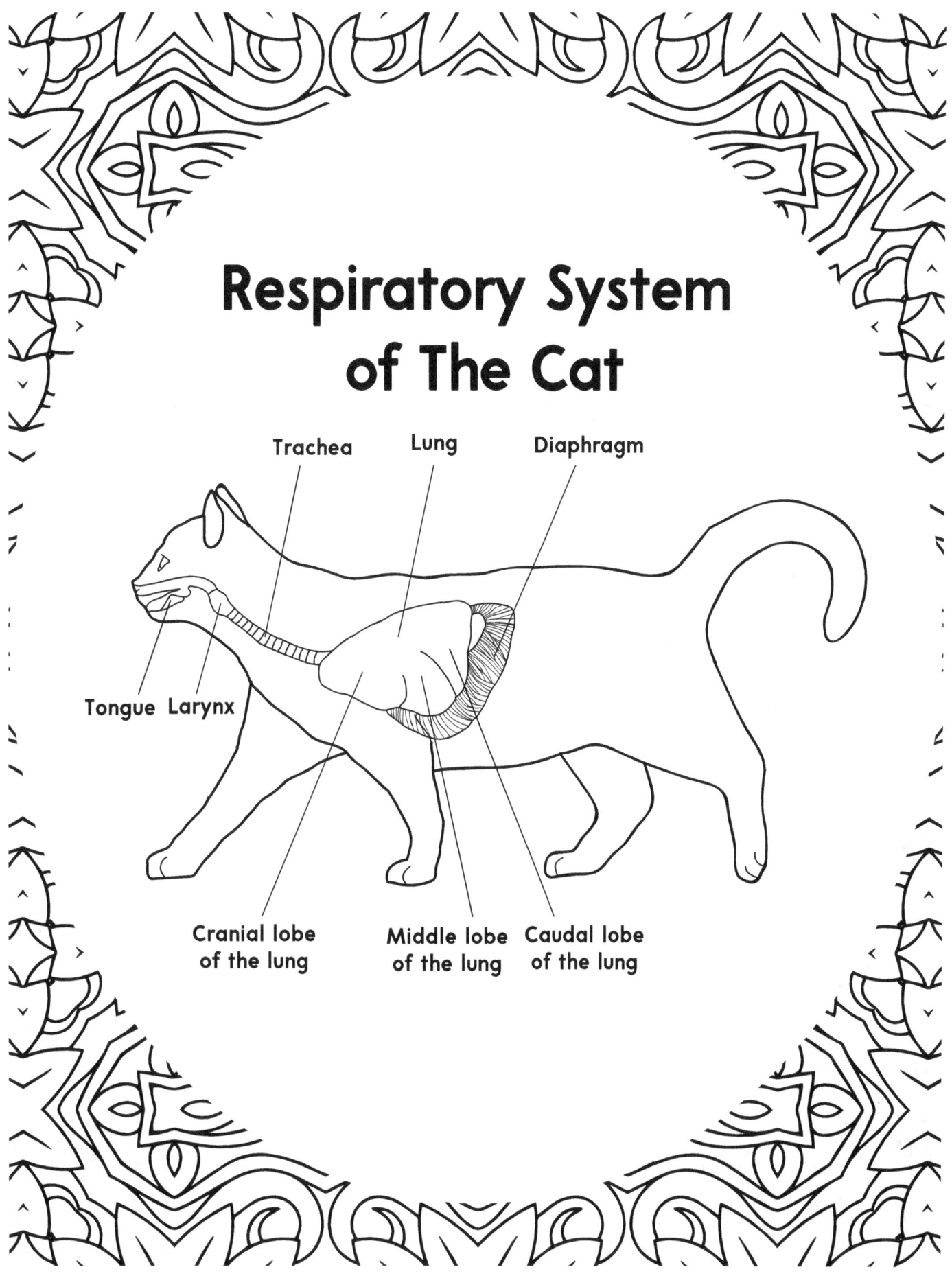

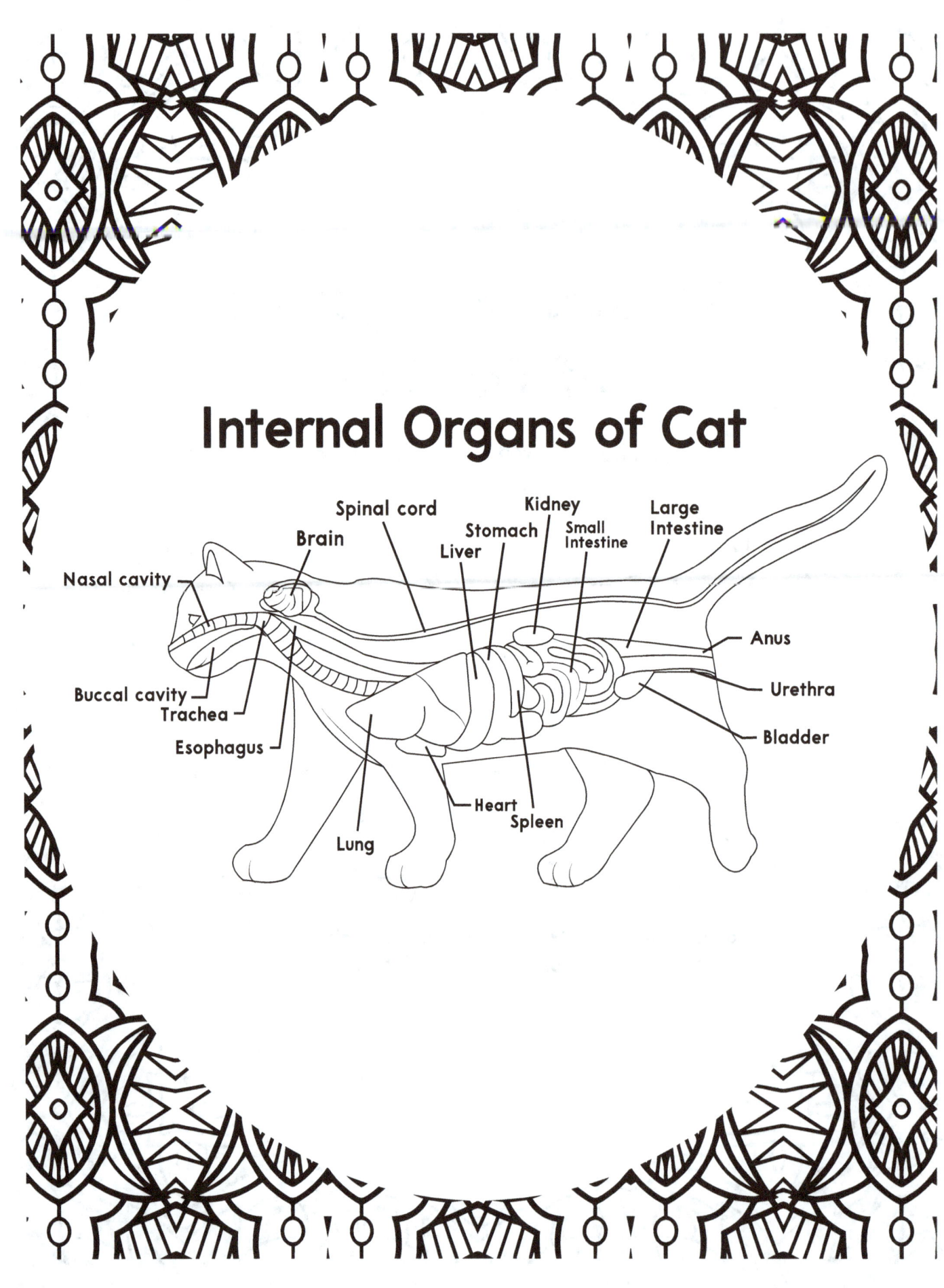

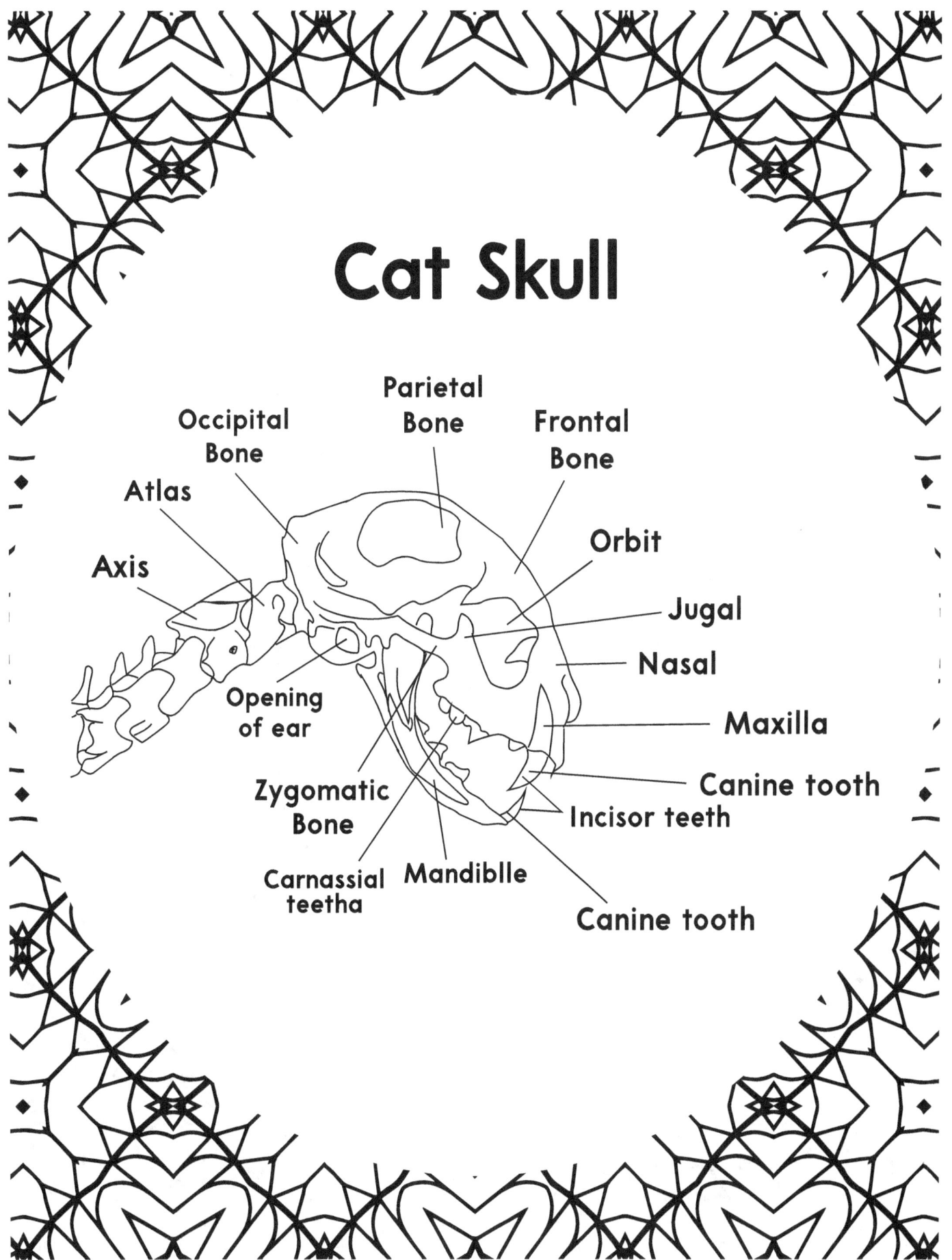

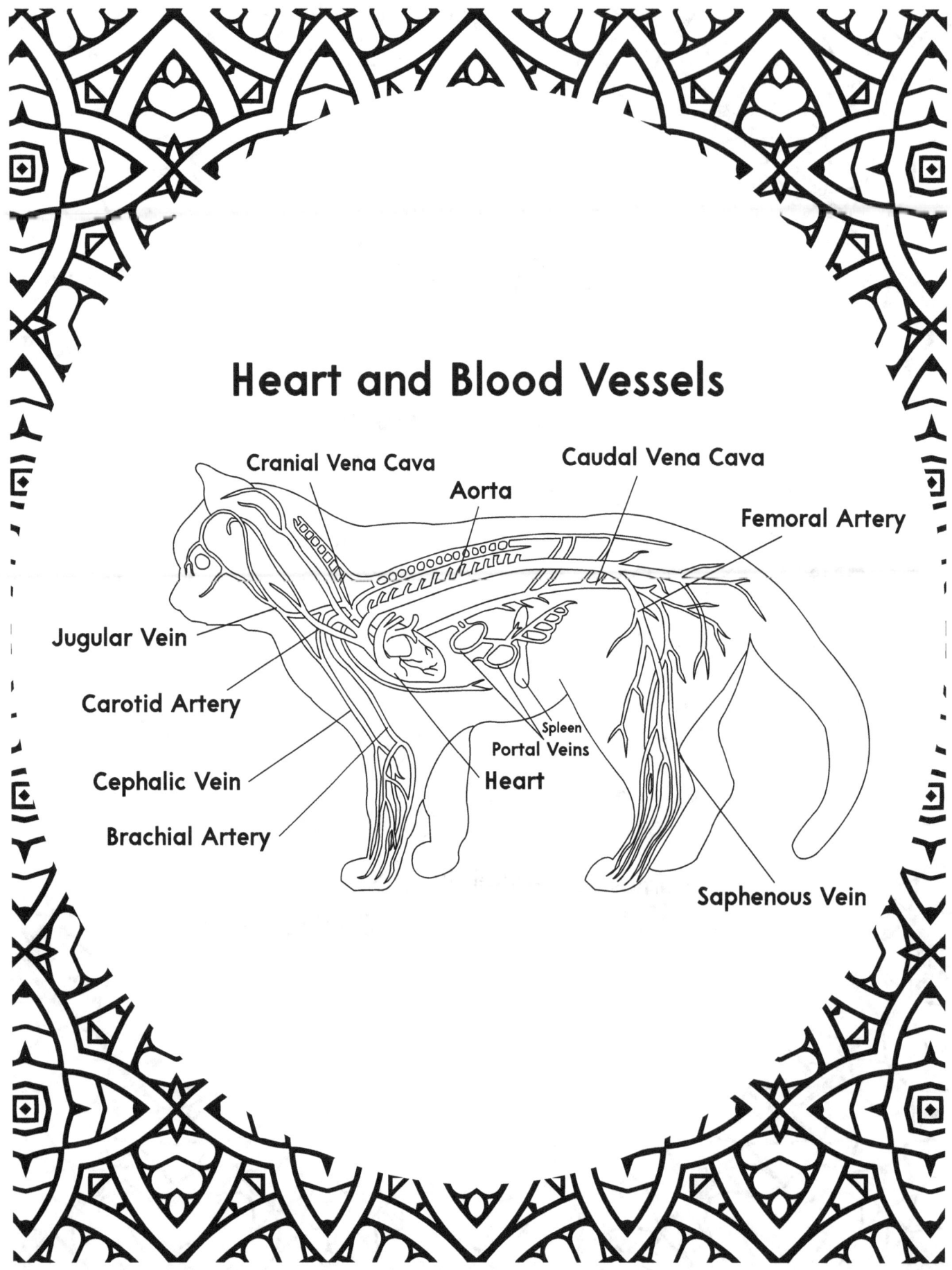

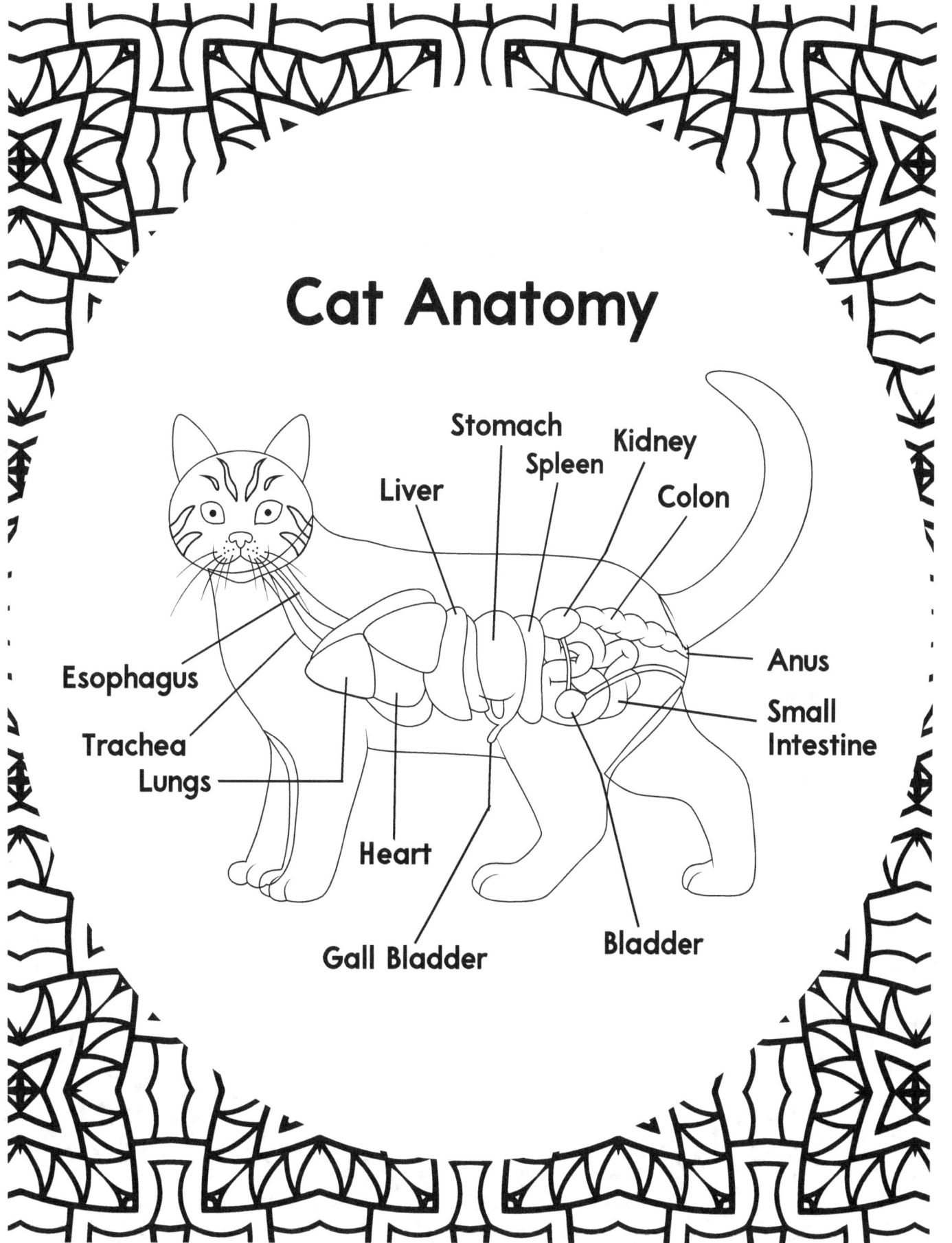

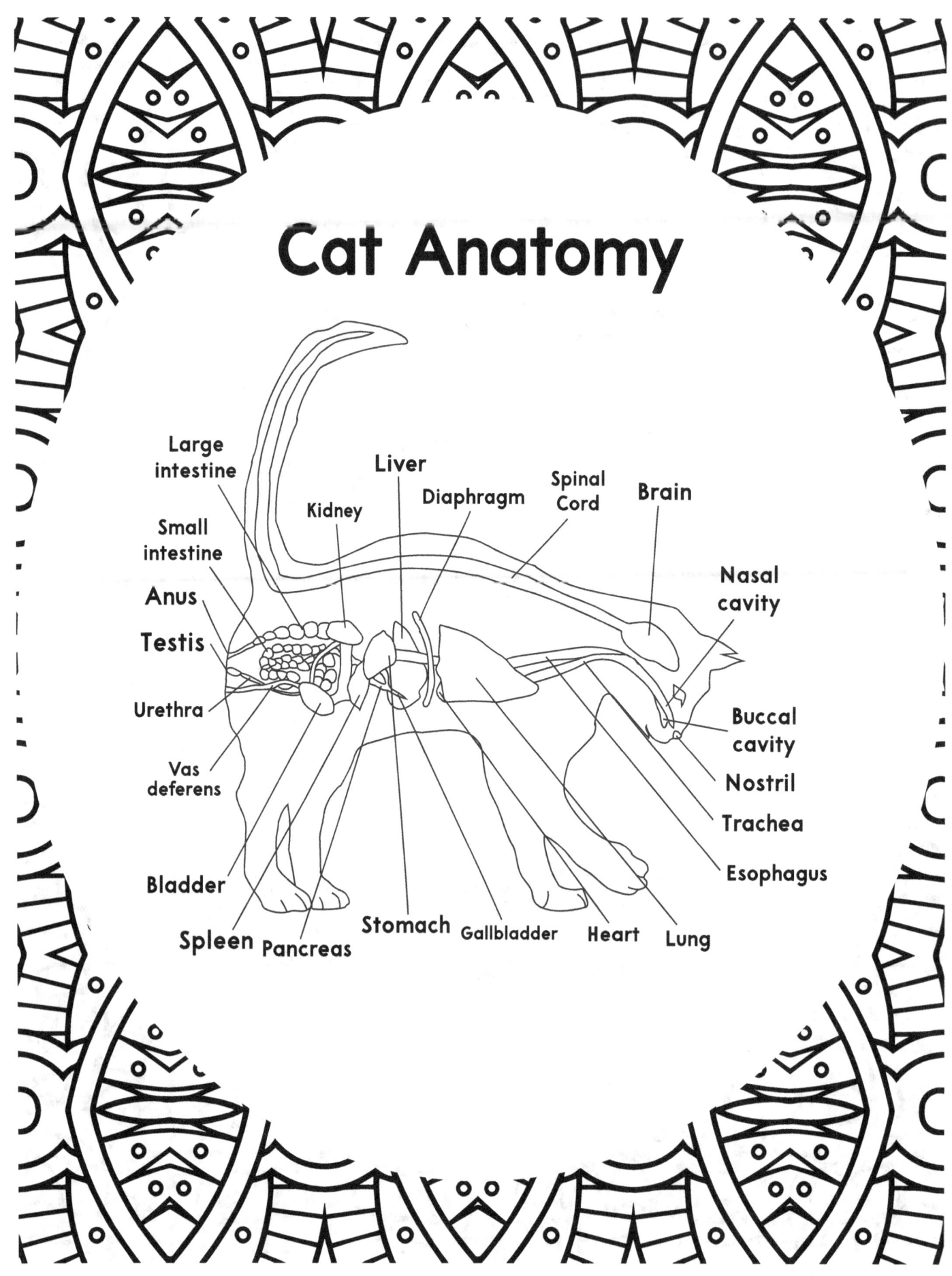

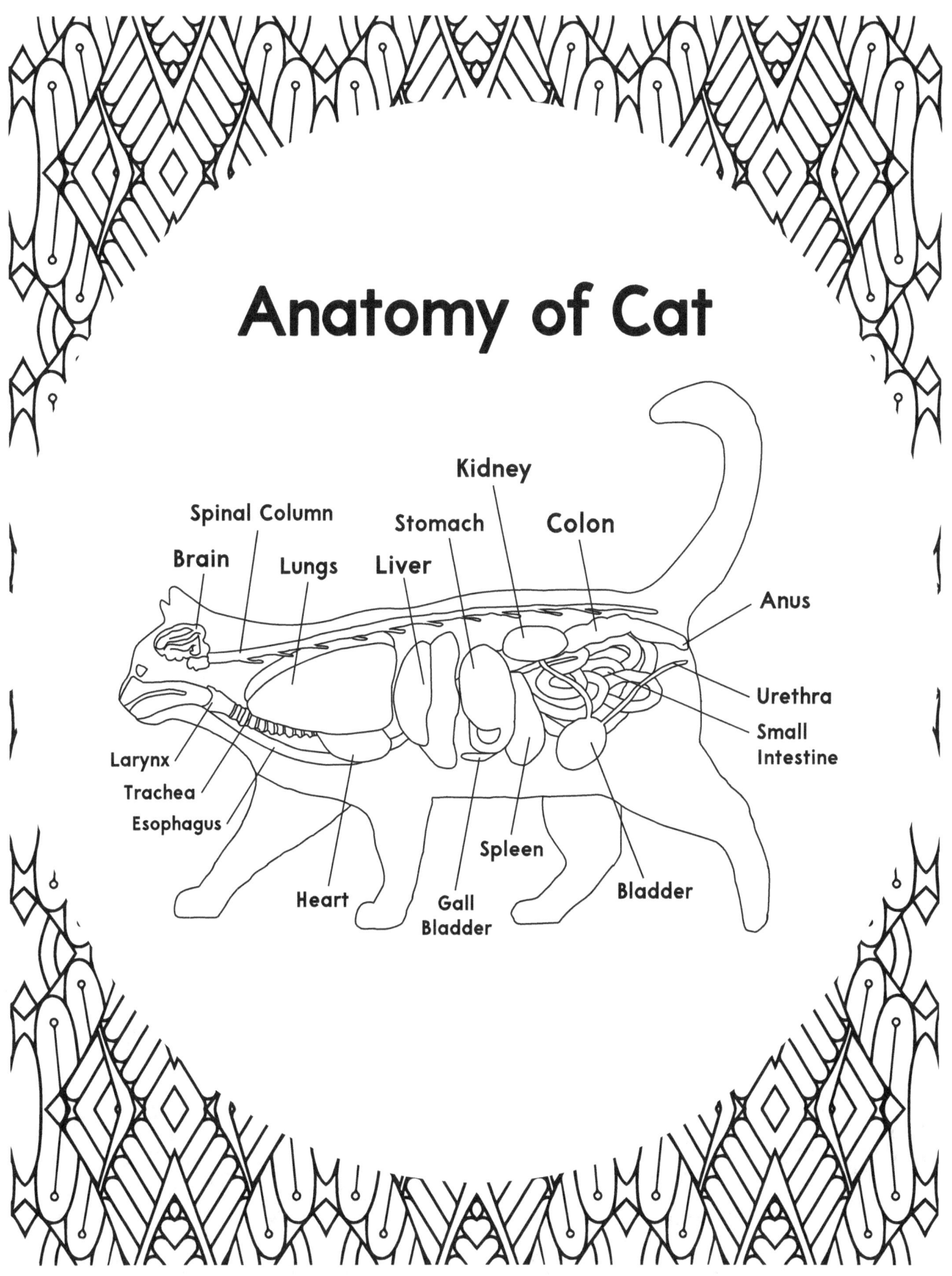

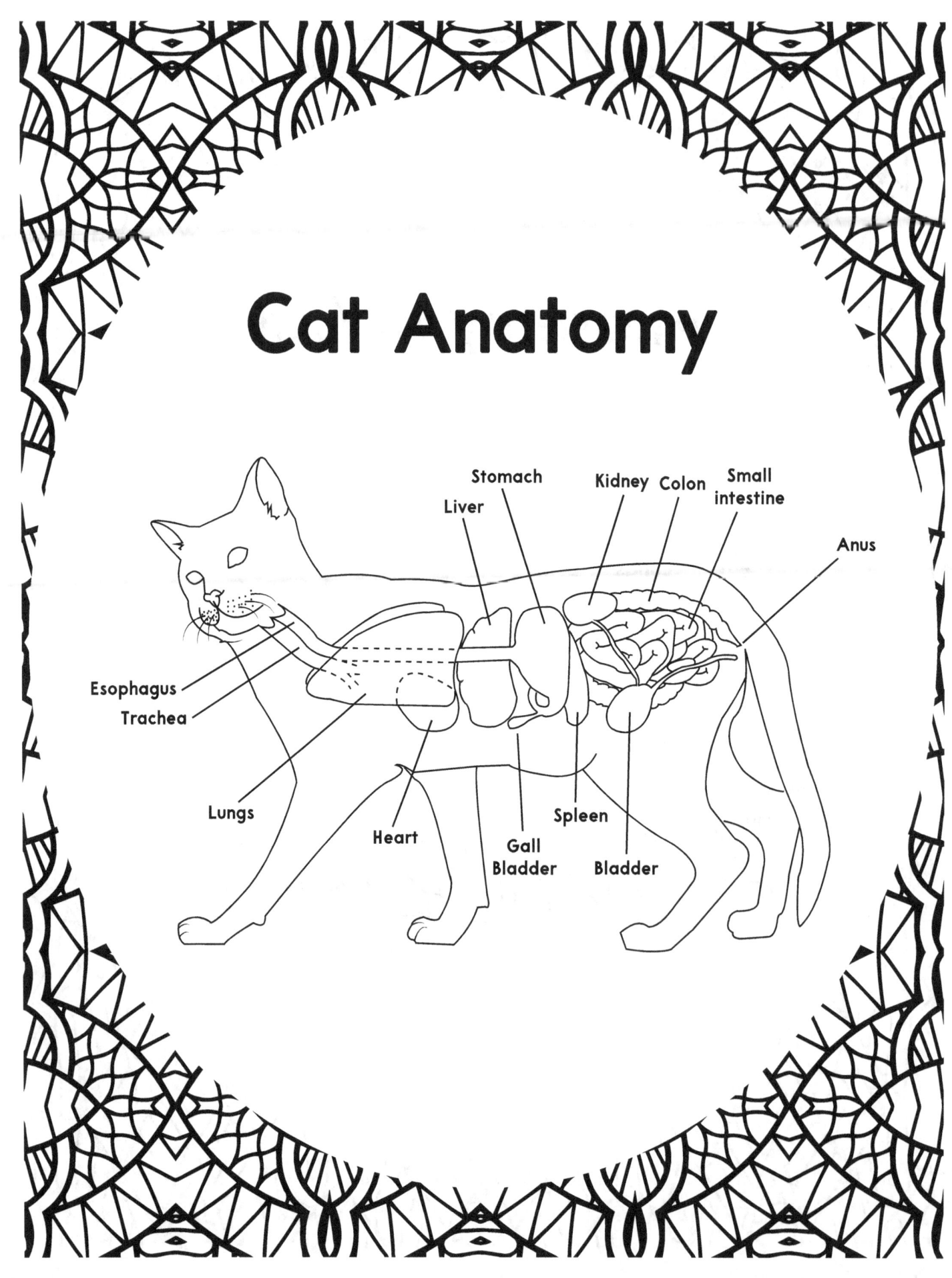

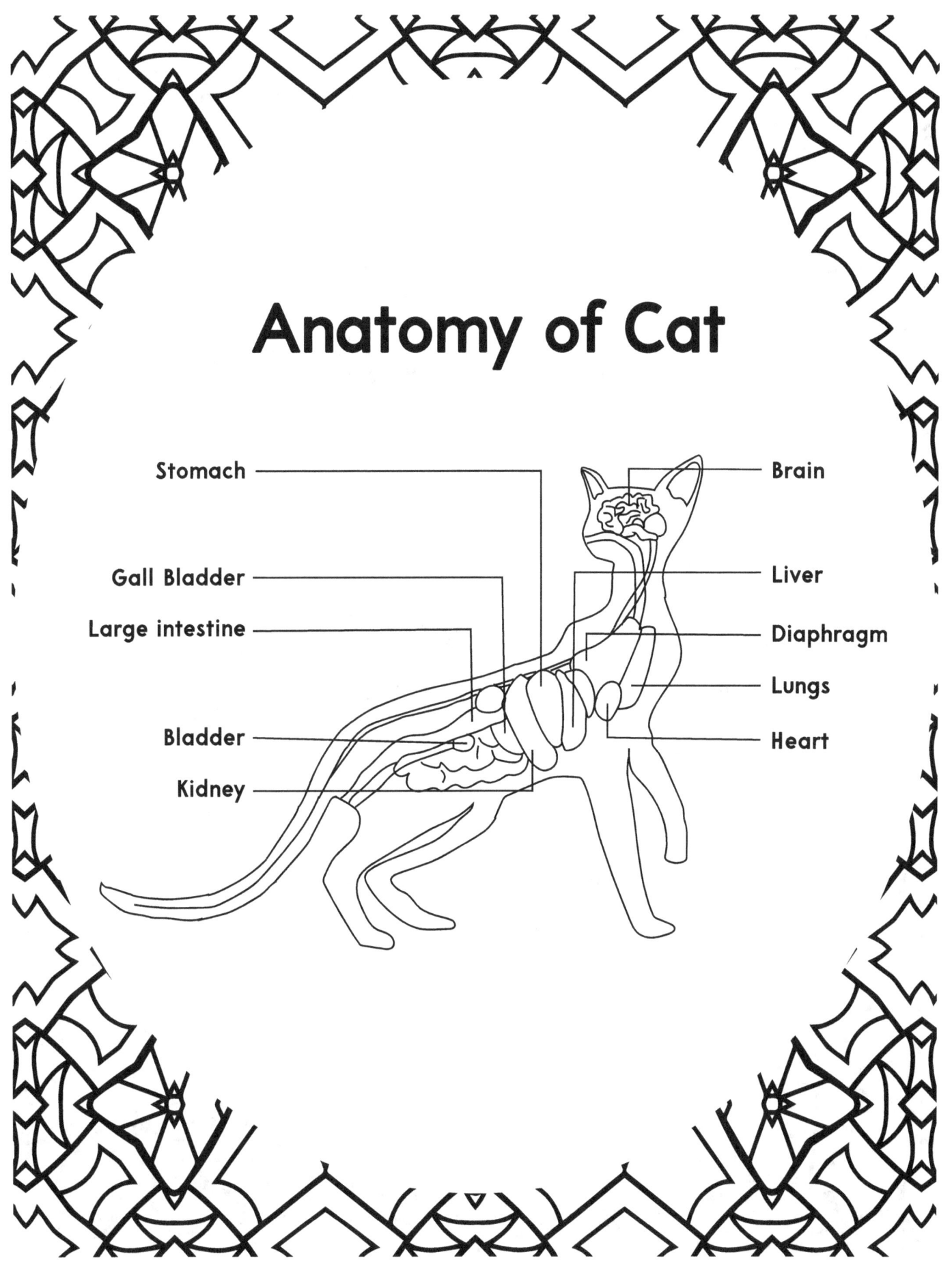

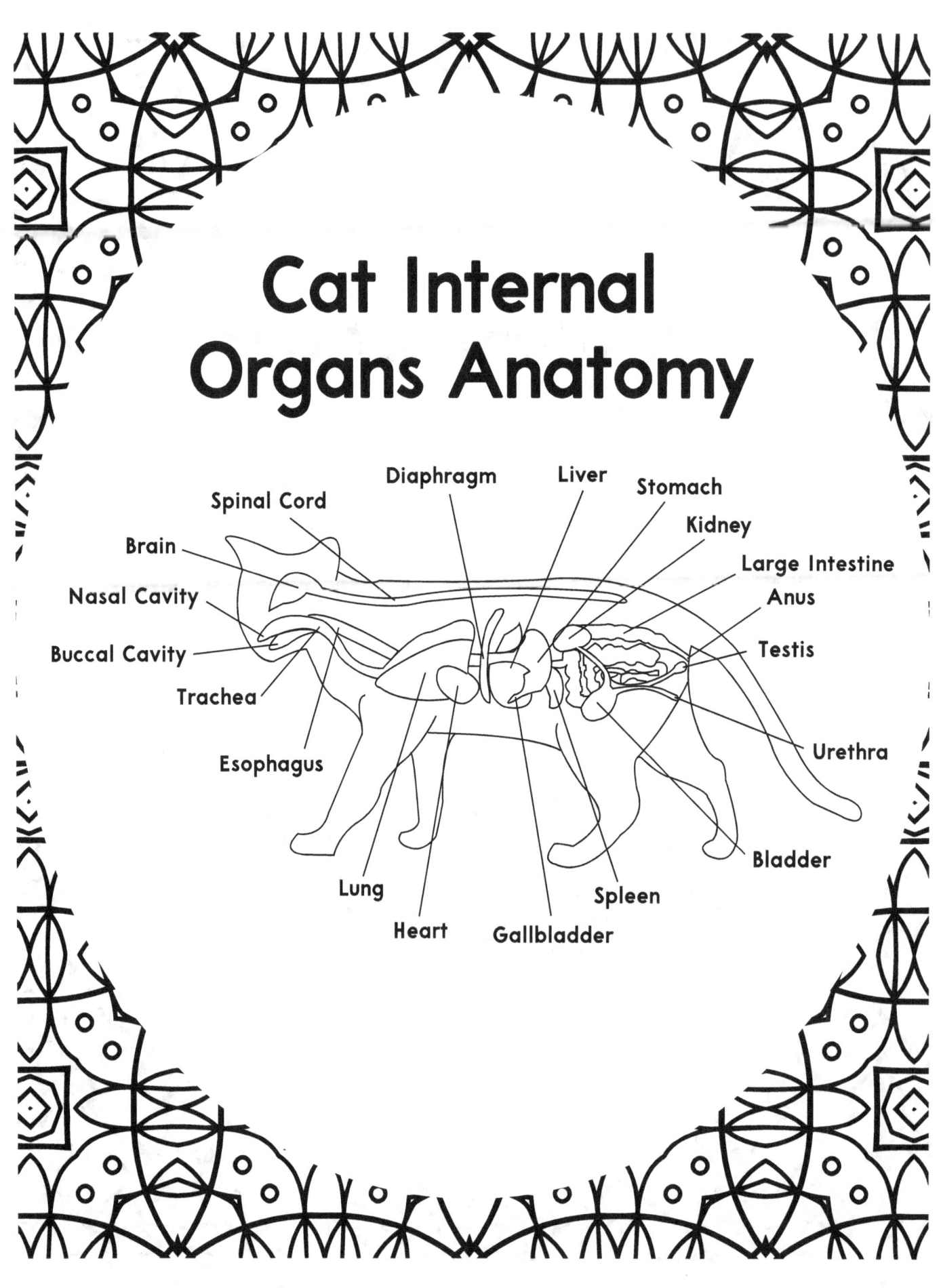

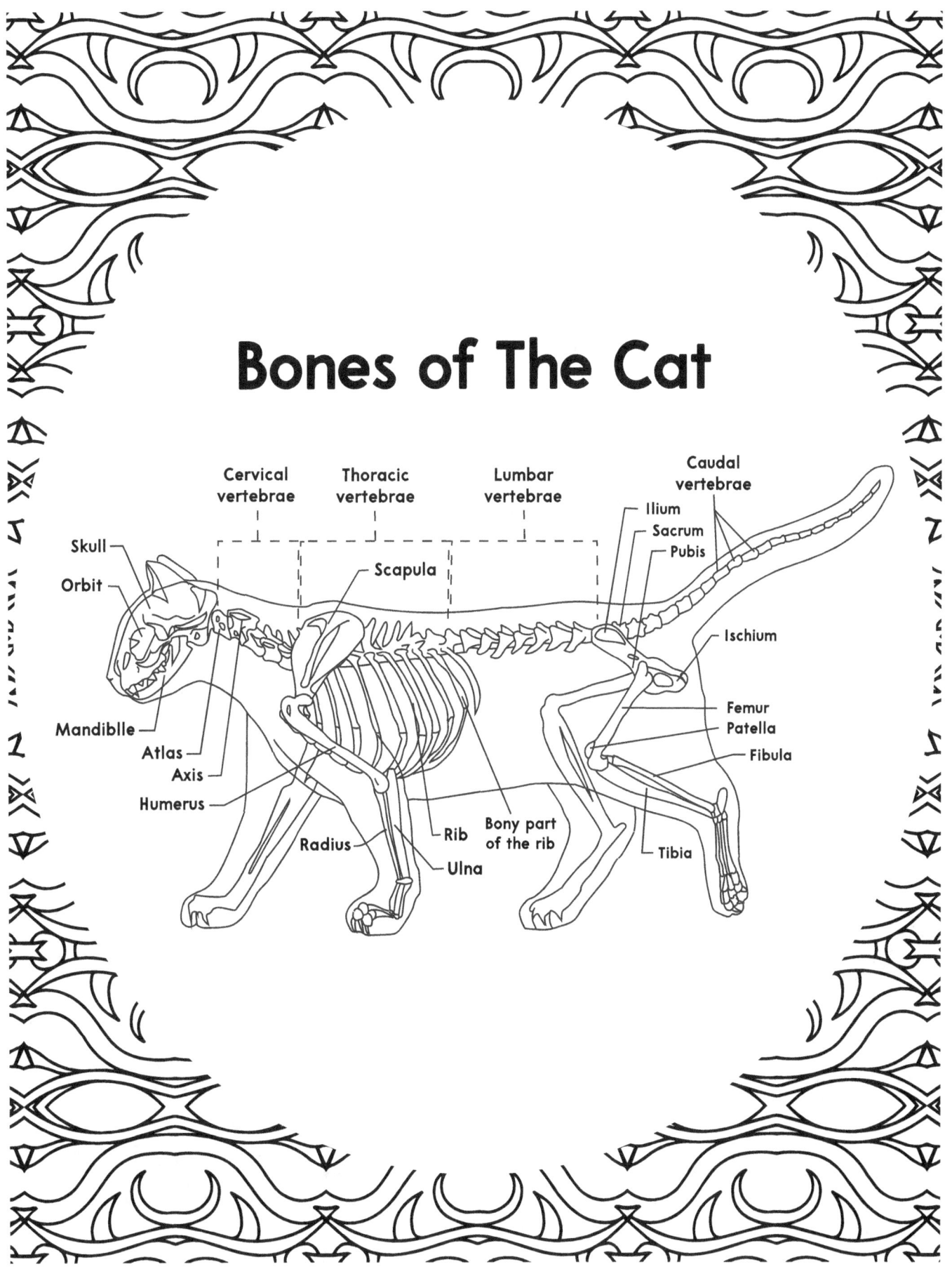

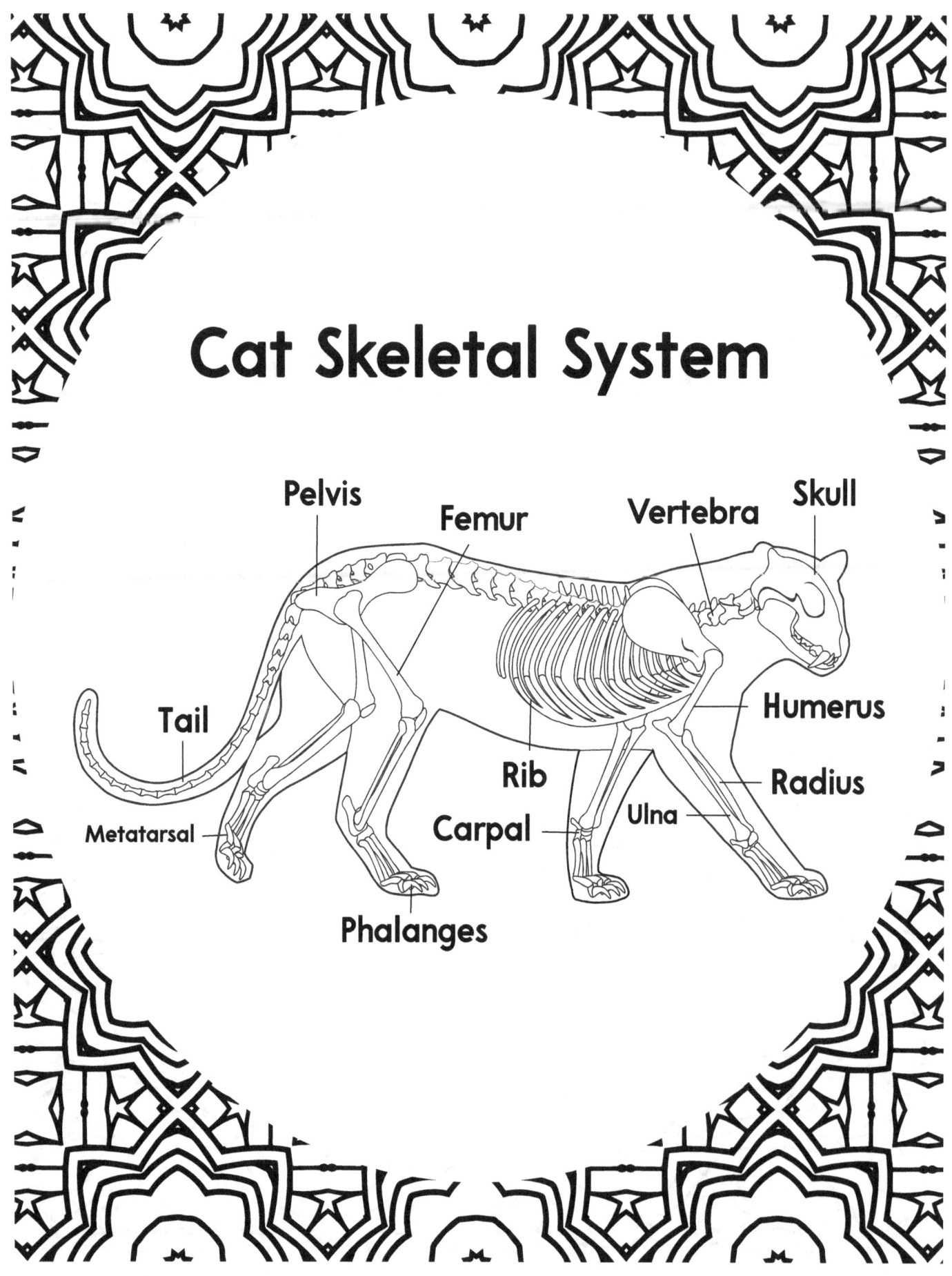

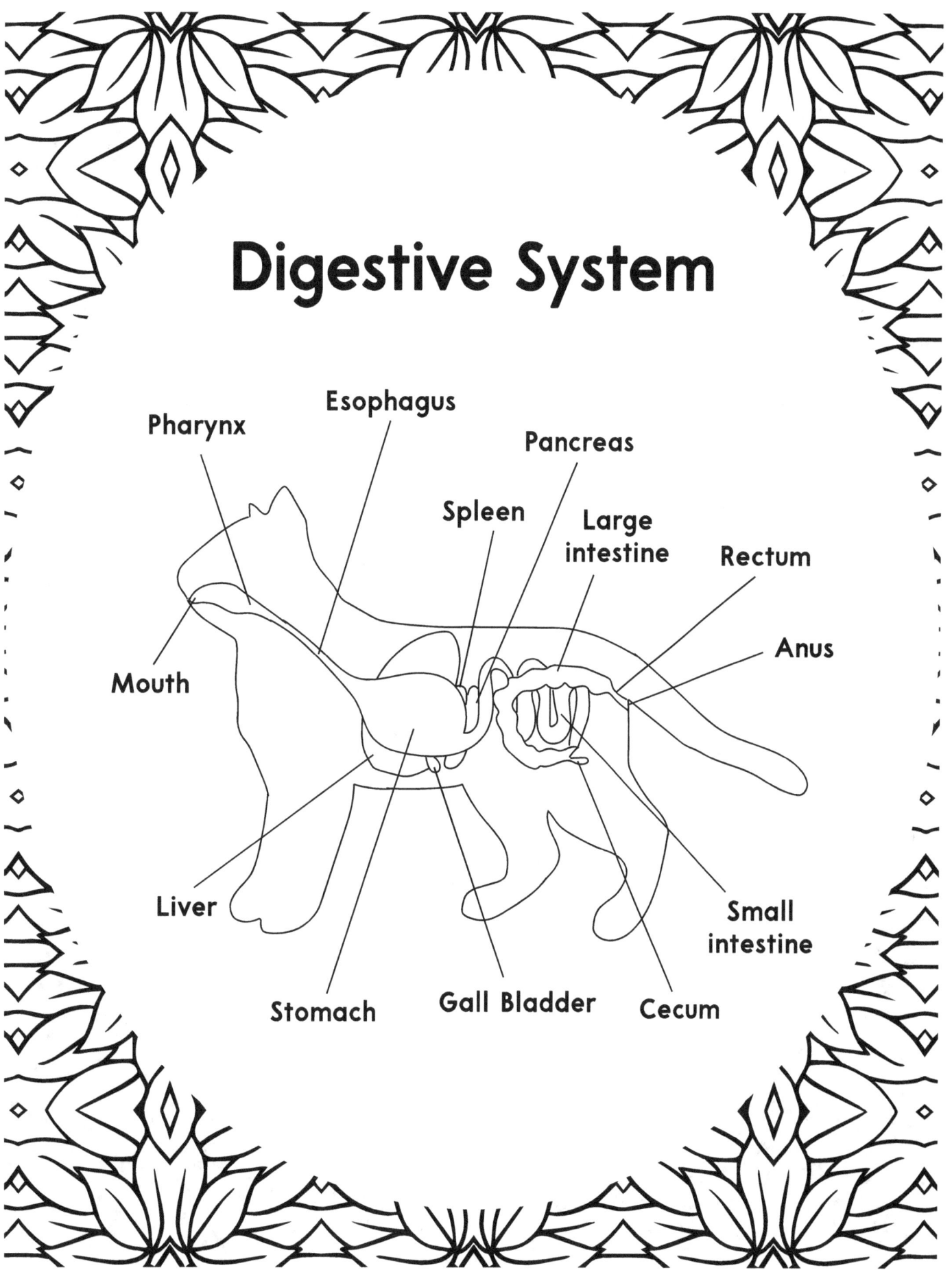

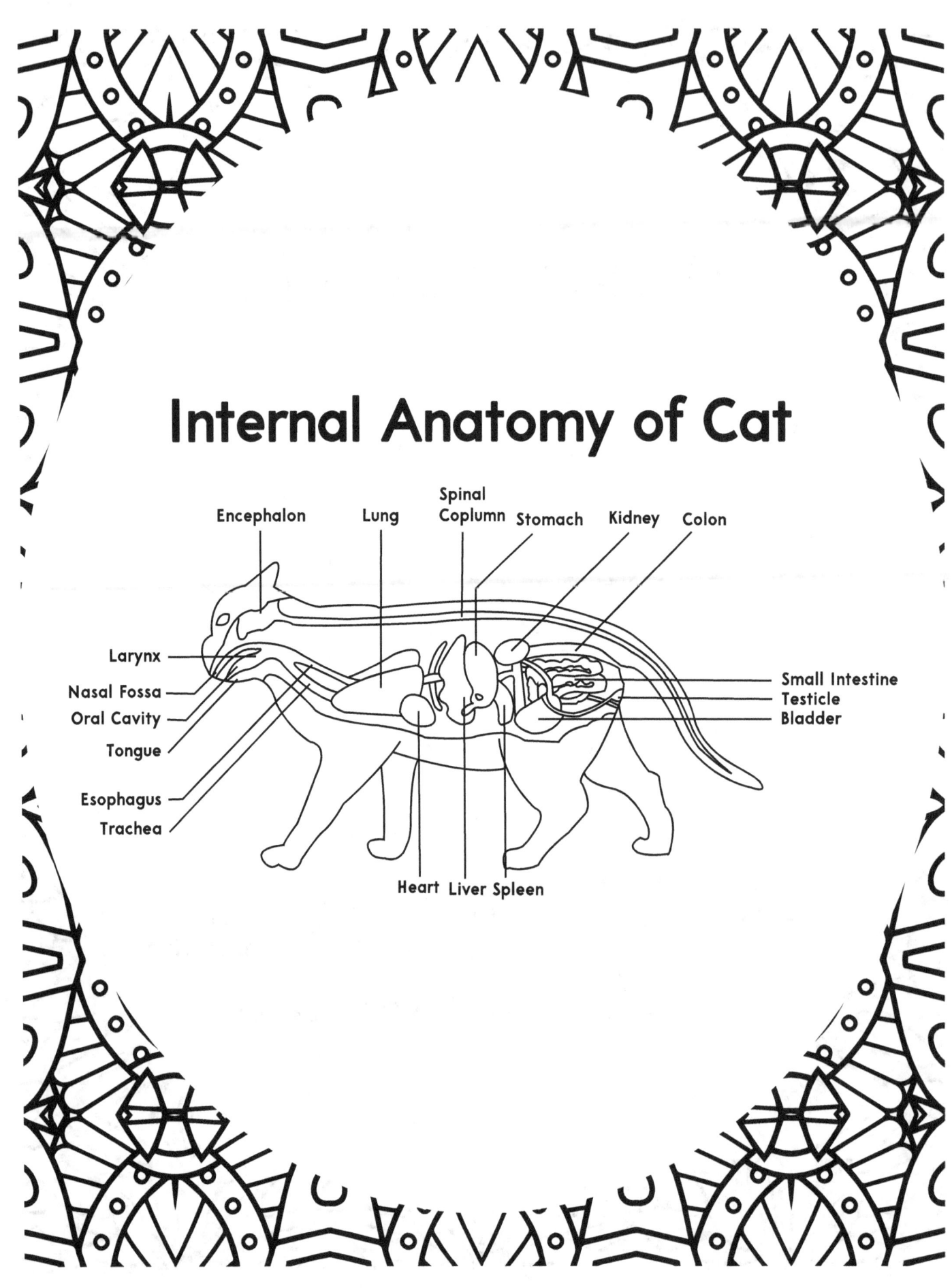

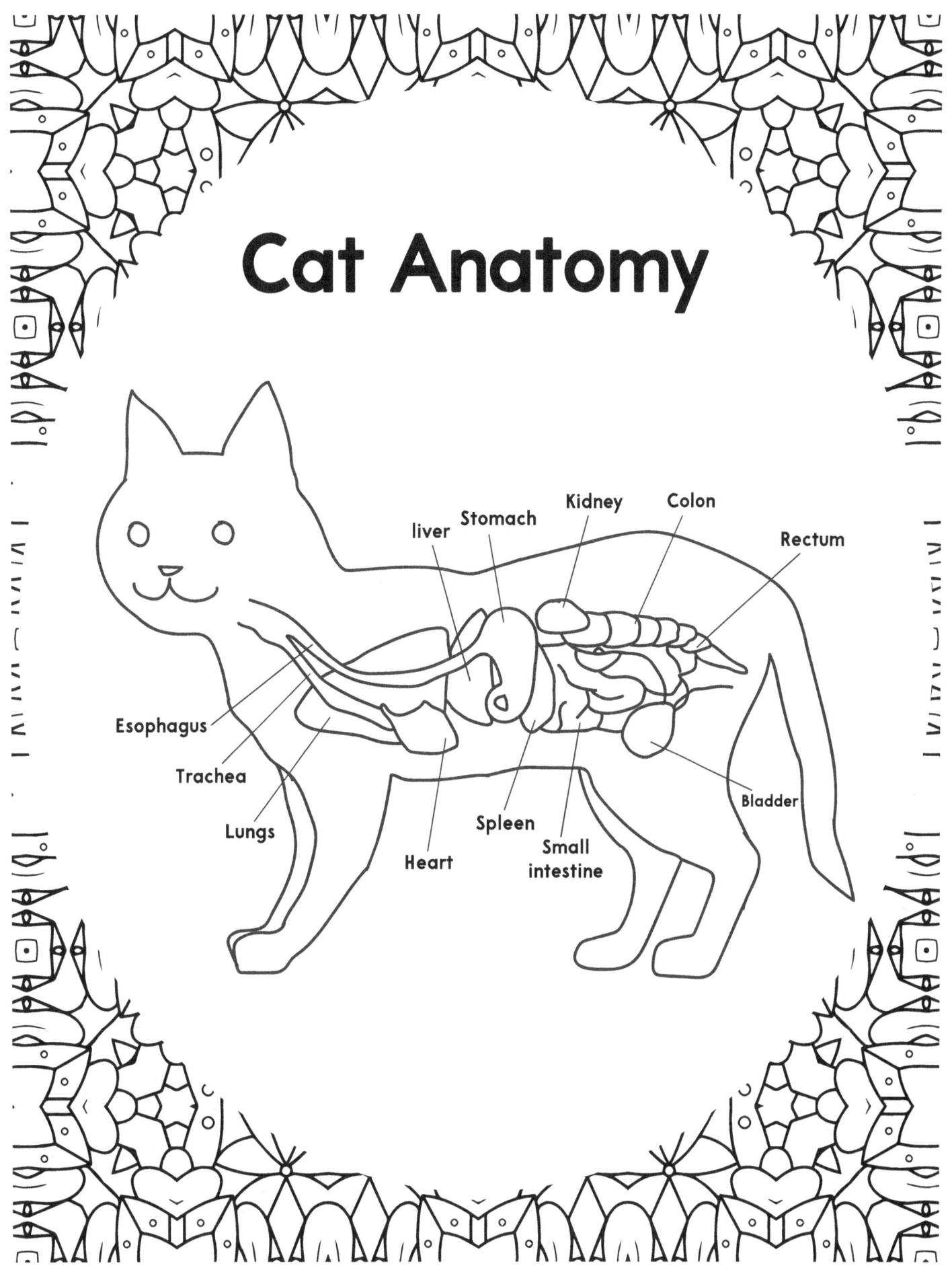

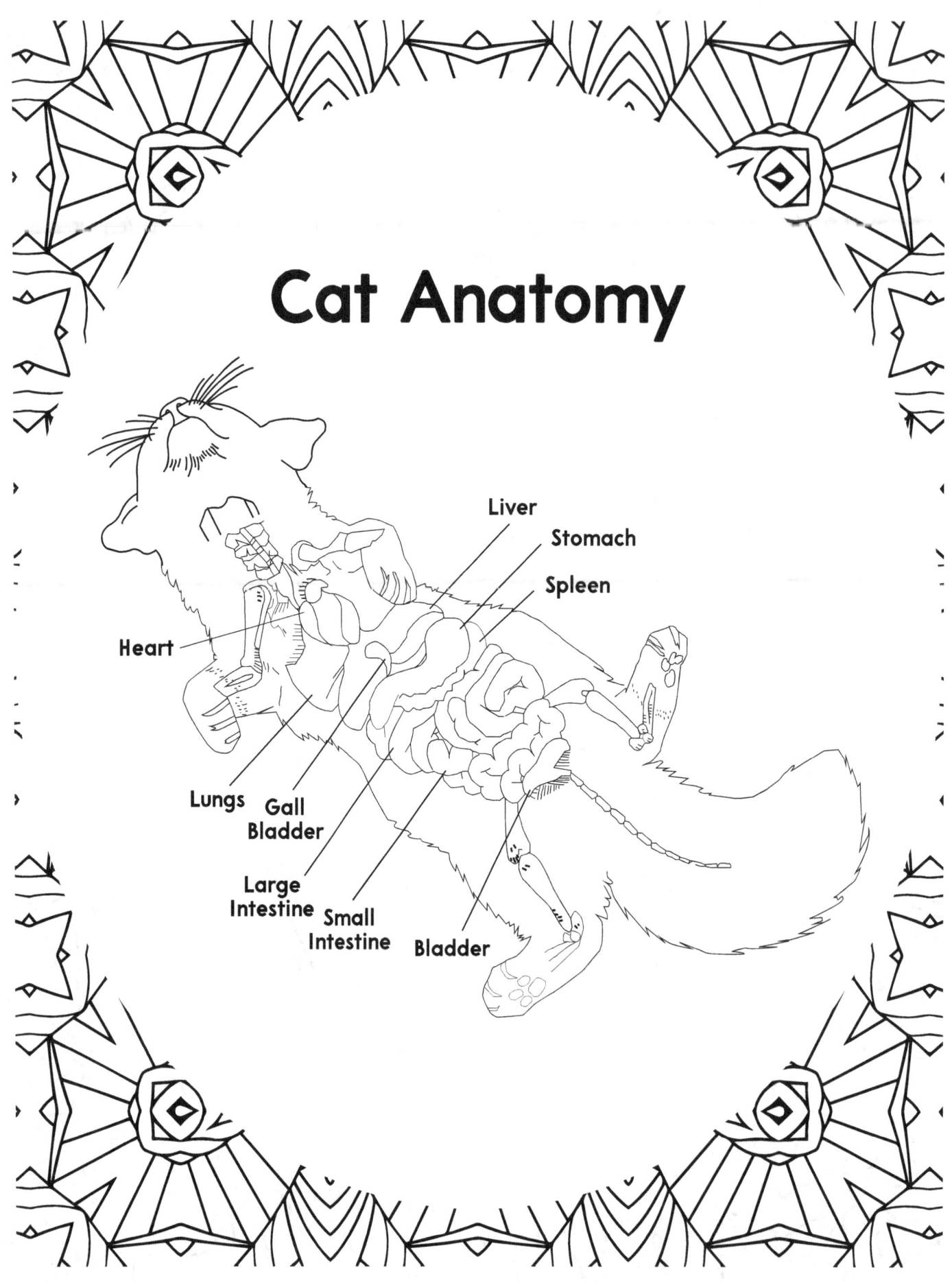

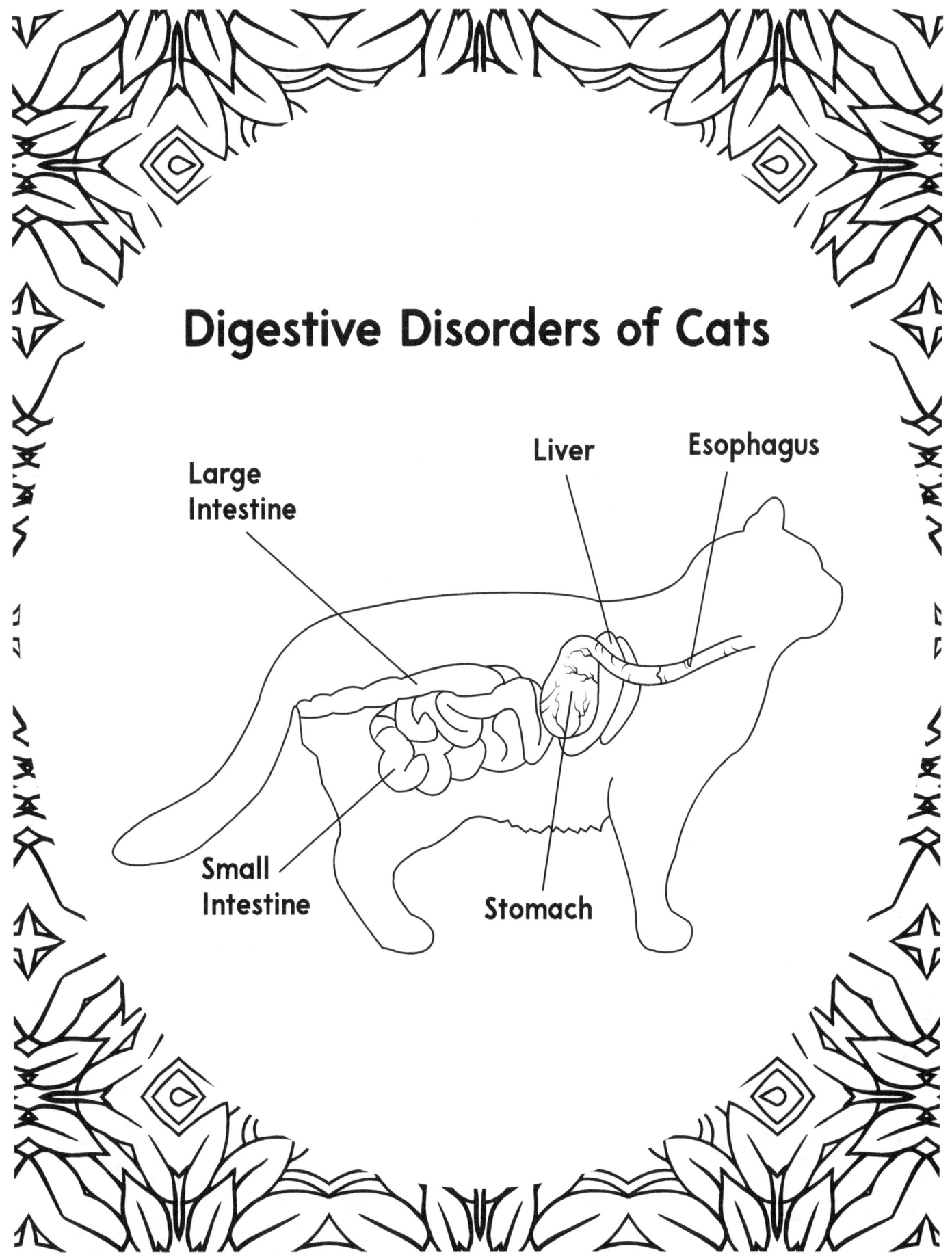

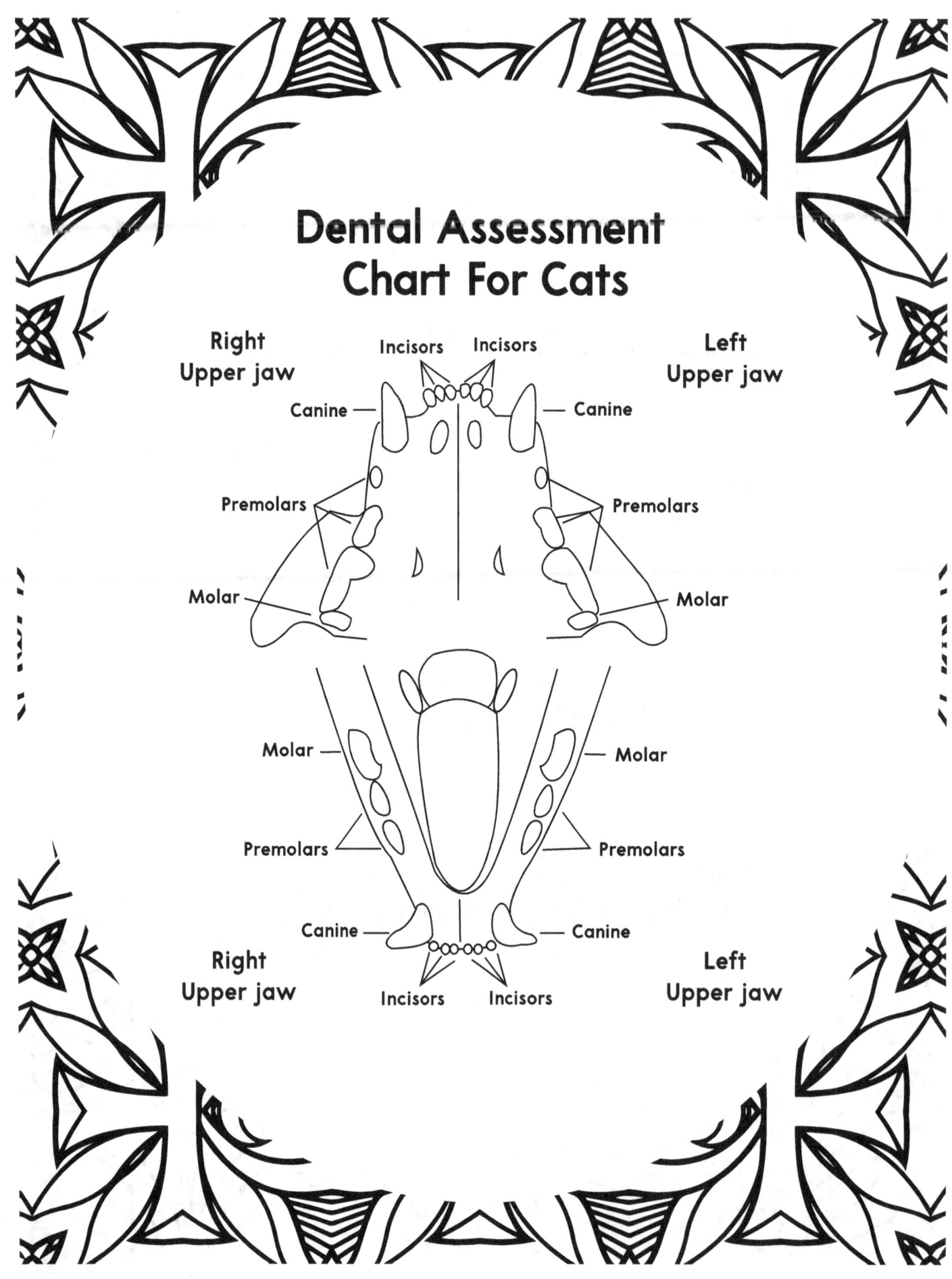

Lymphatic System

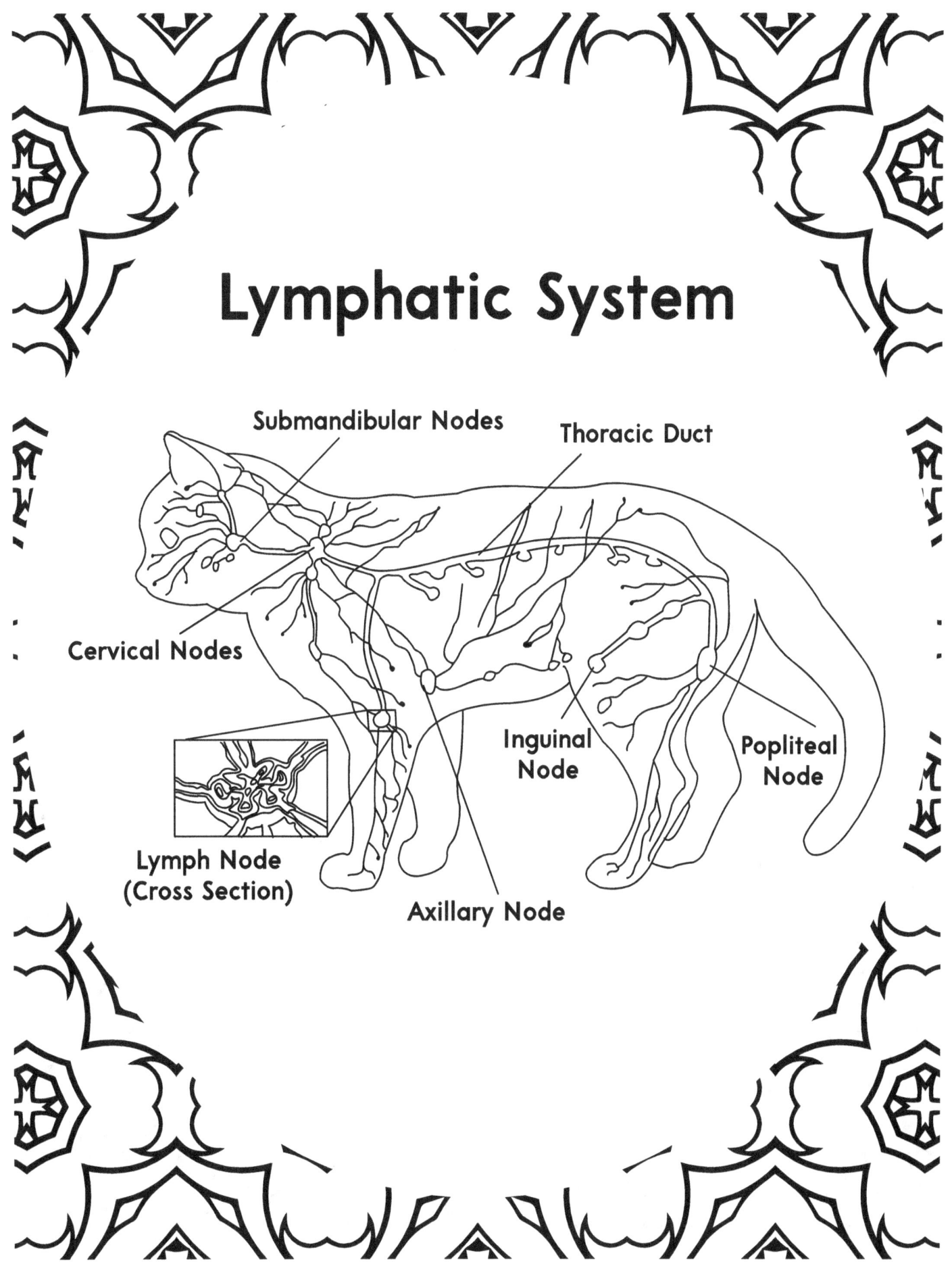

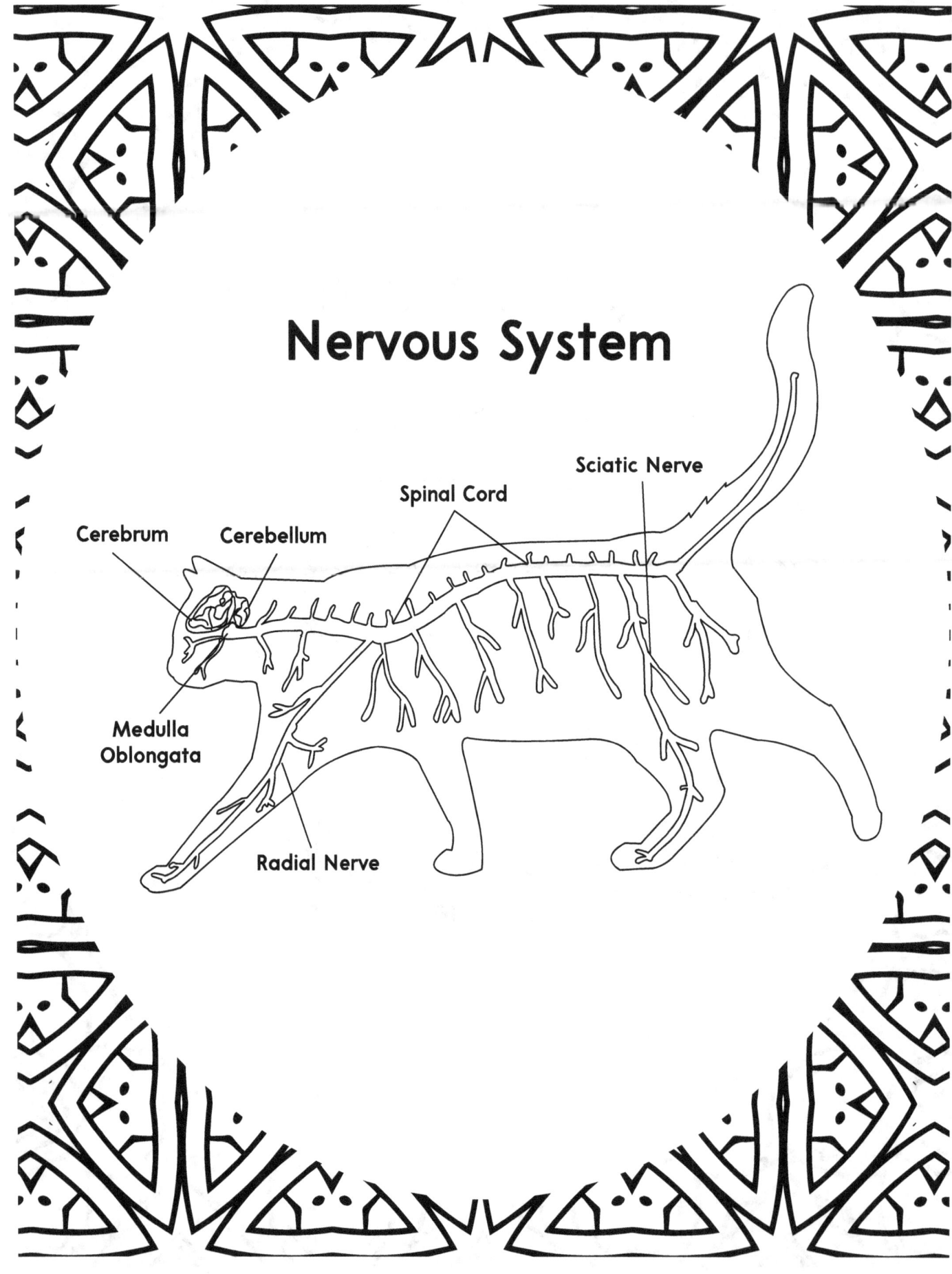

Respiratory System

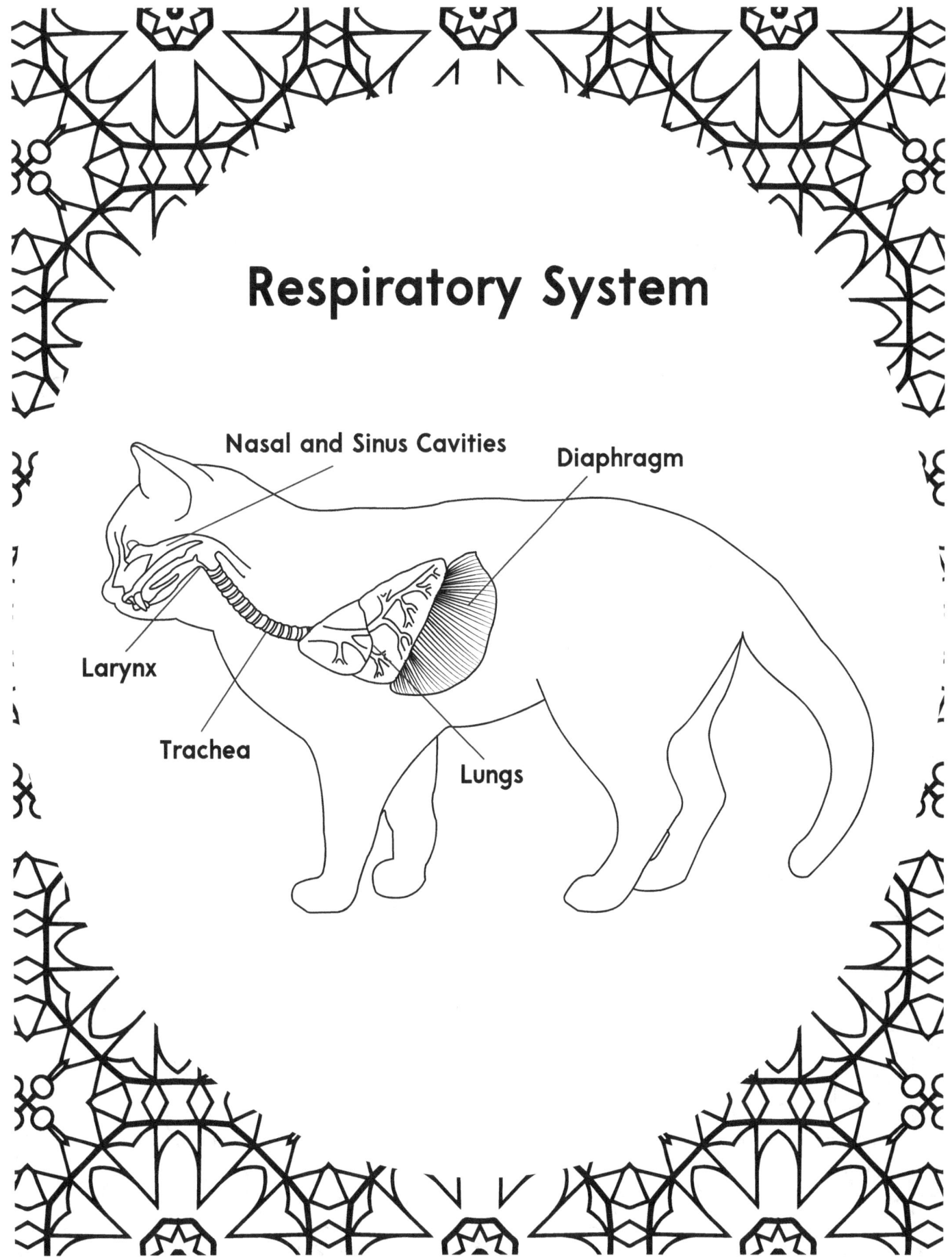

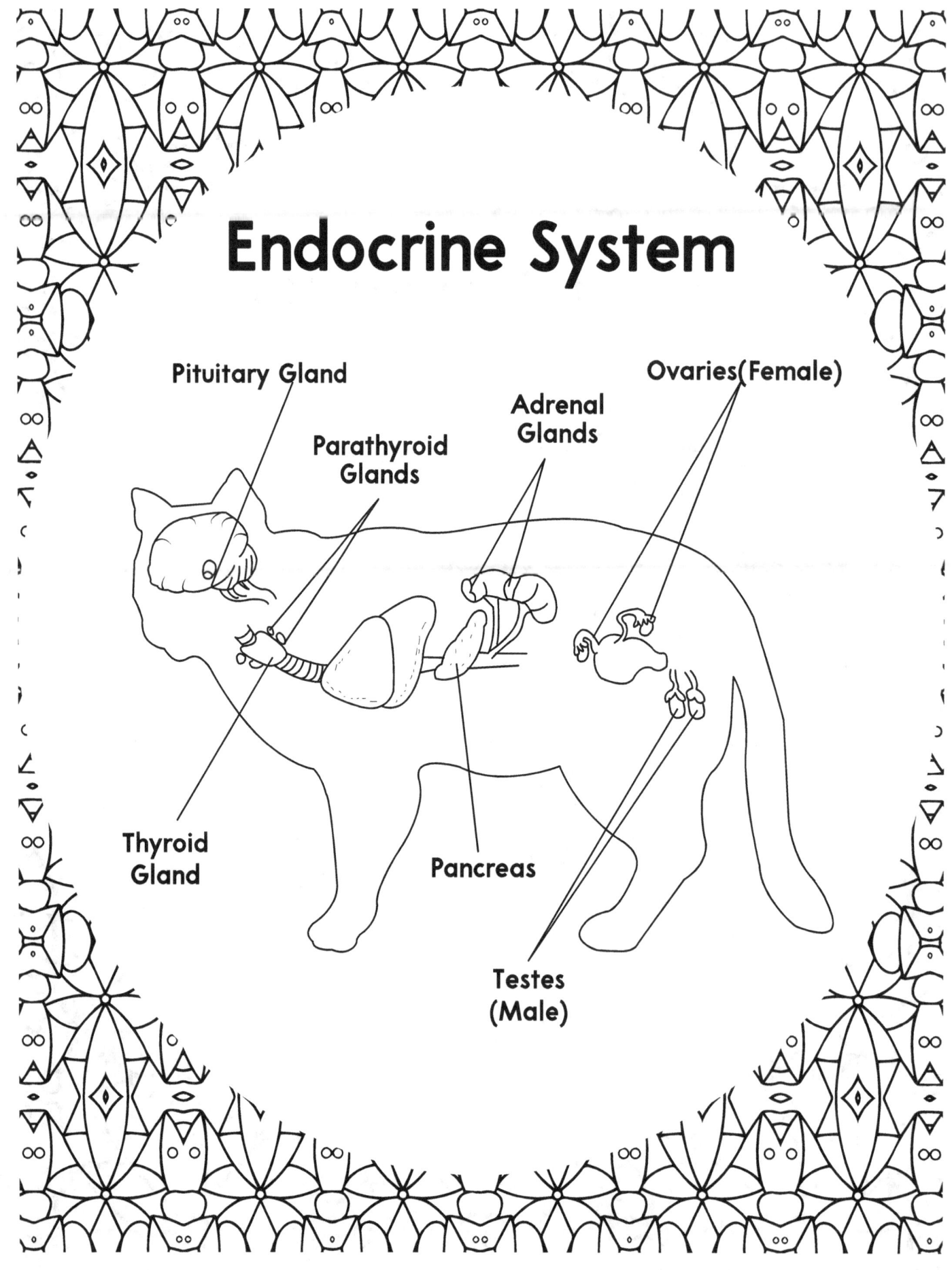

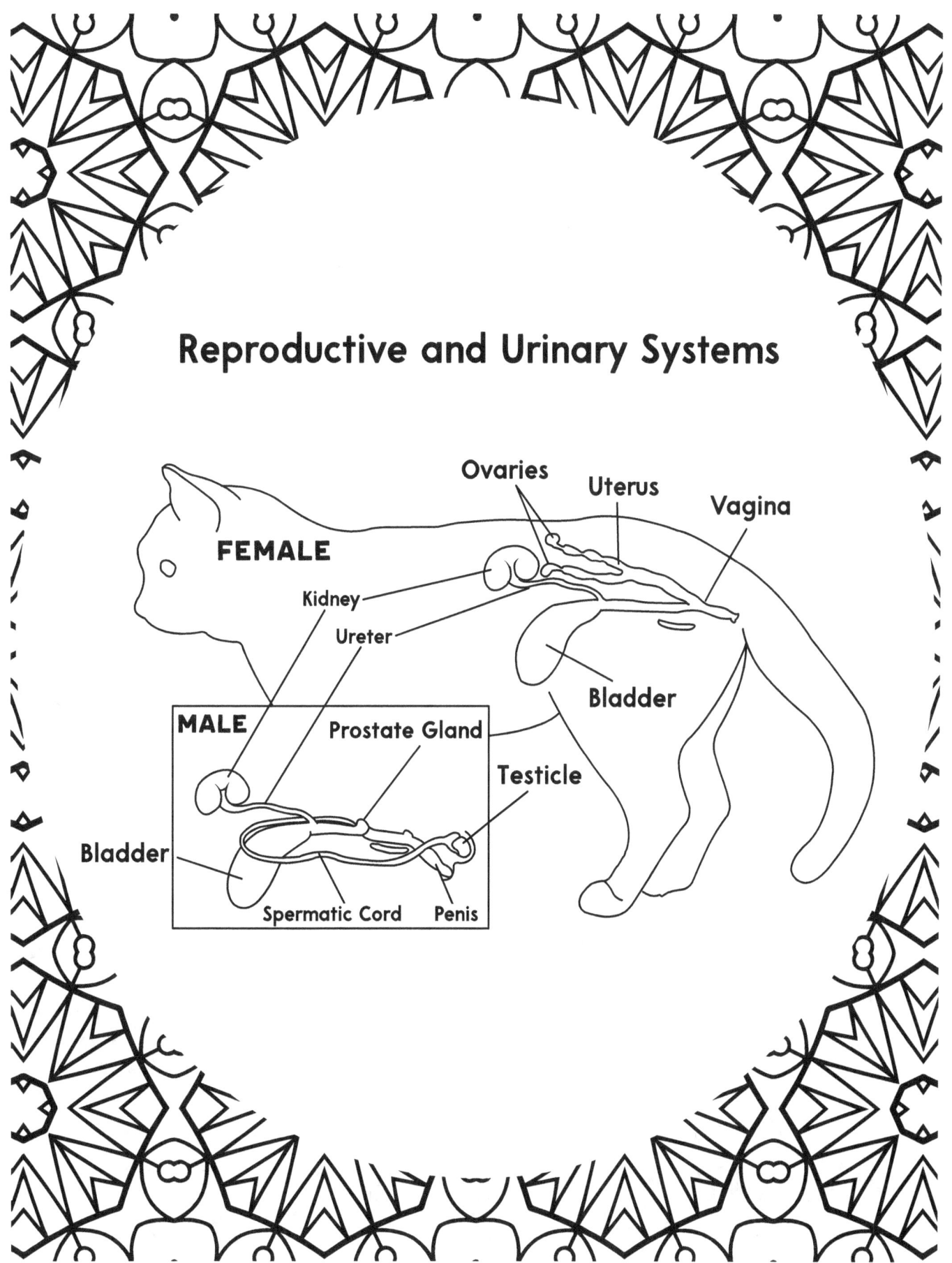

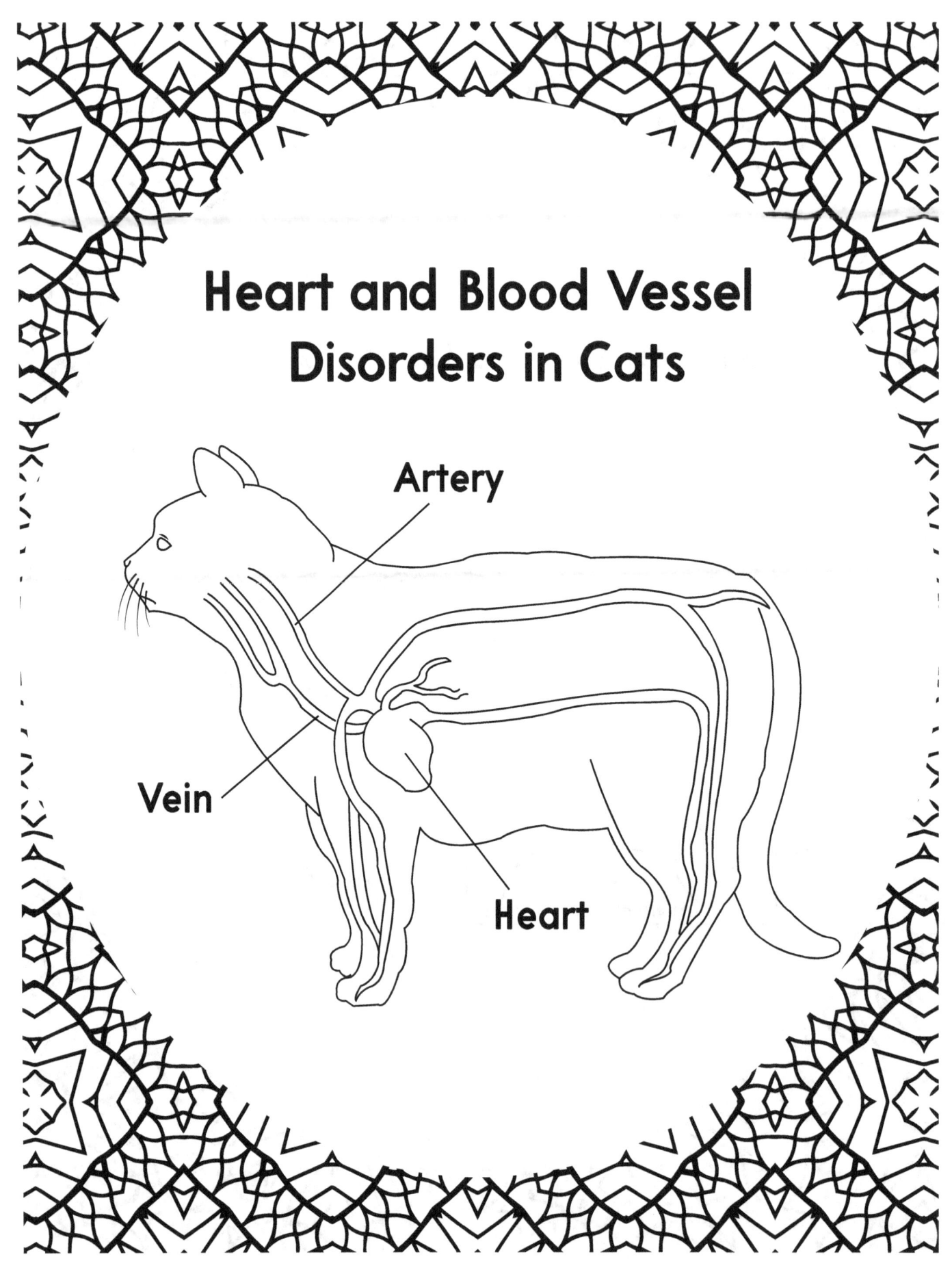

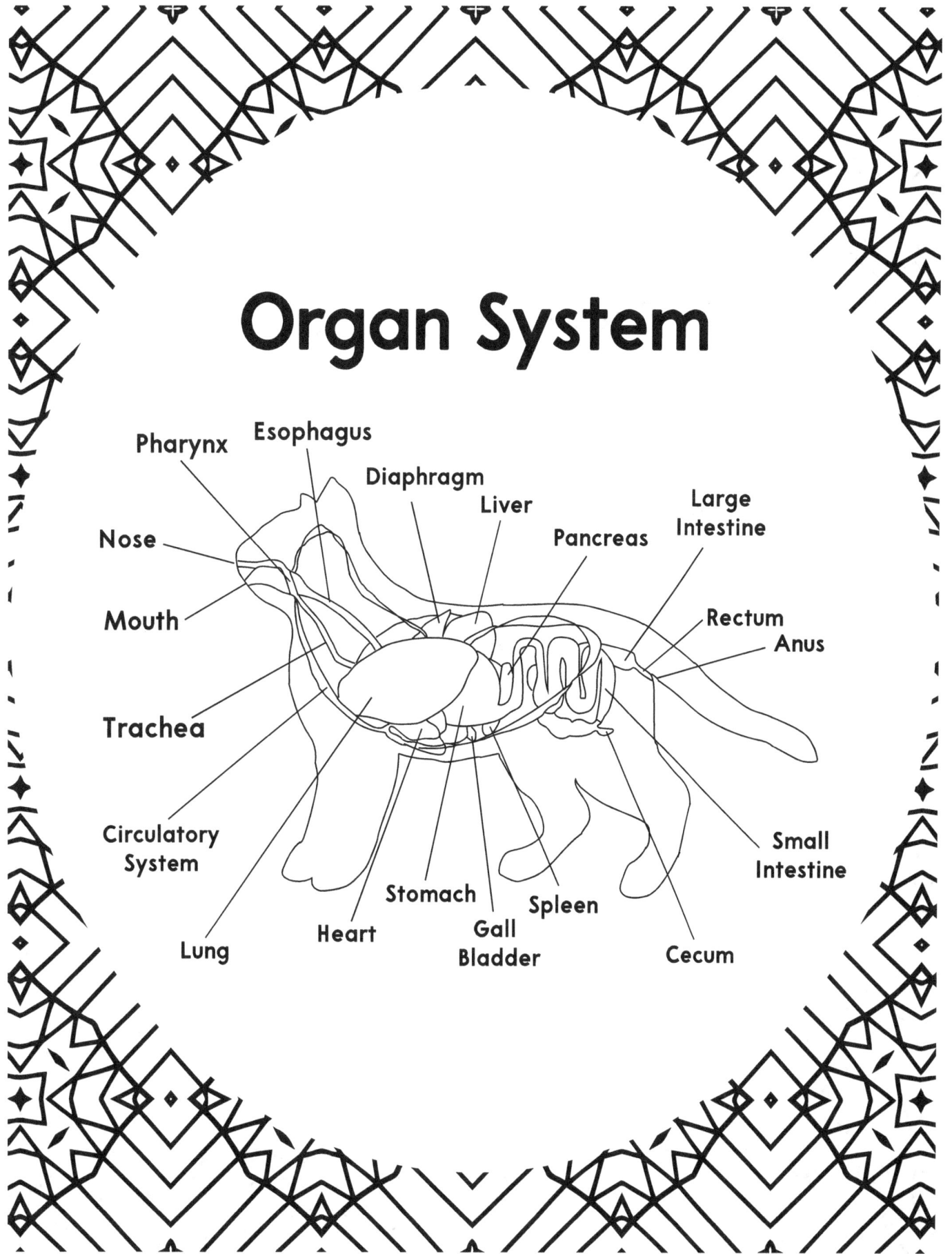

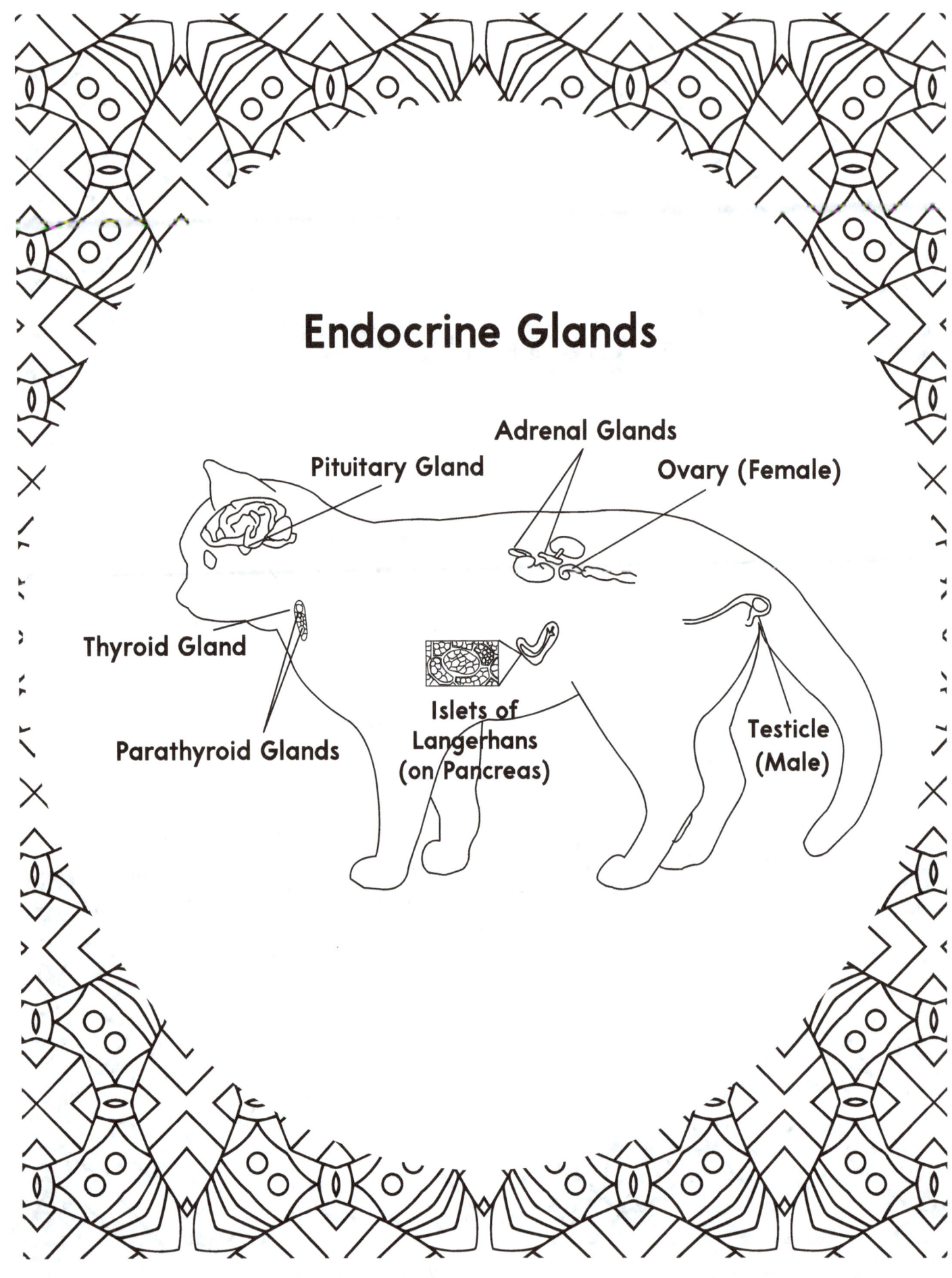

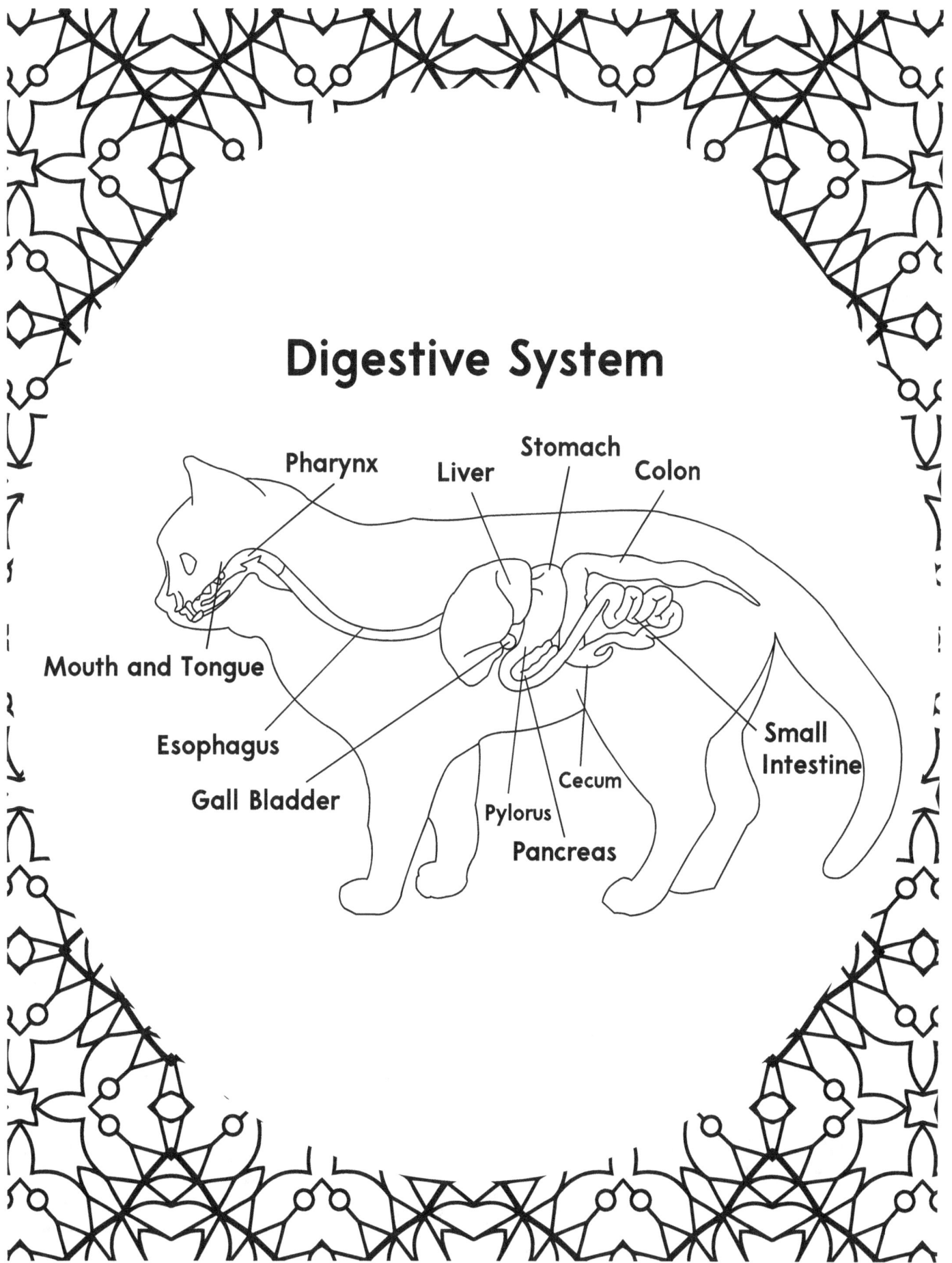

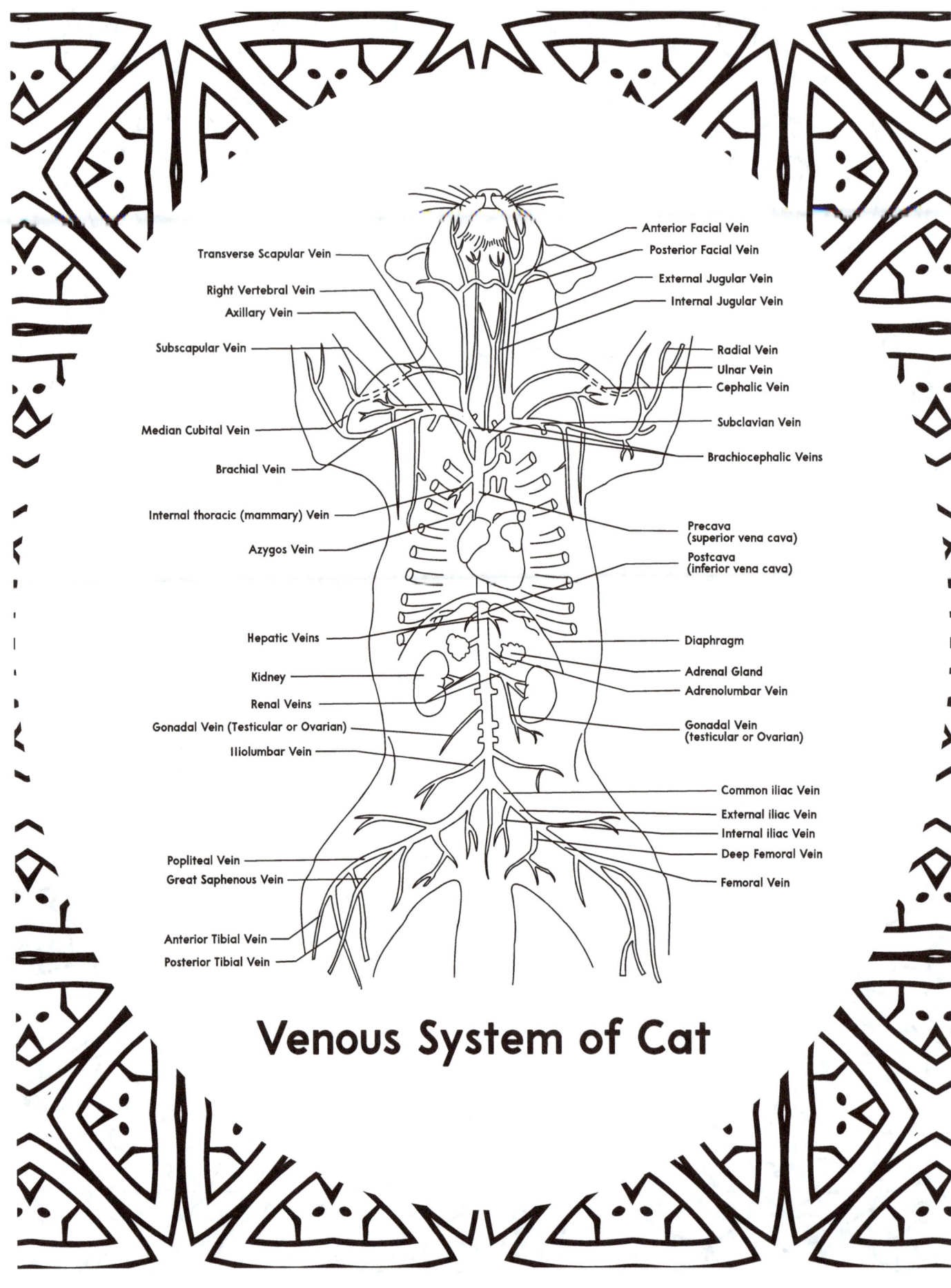

Reproductive System

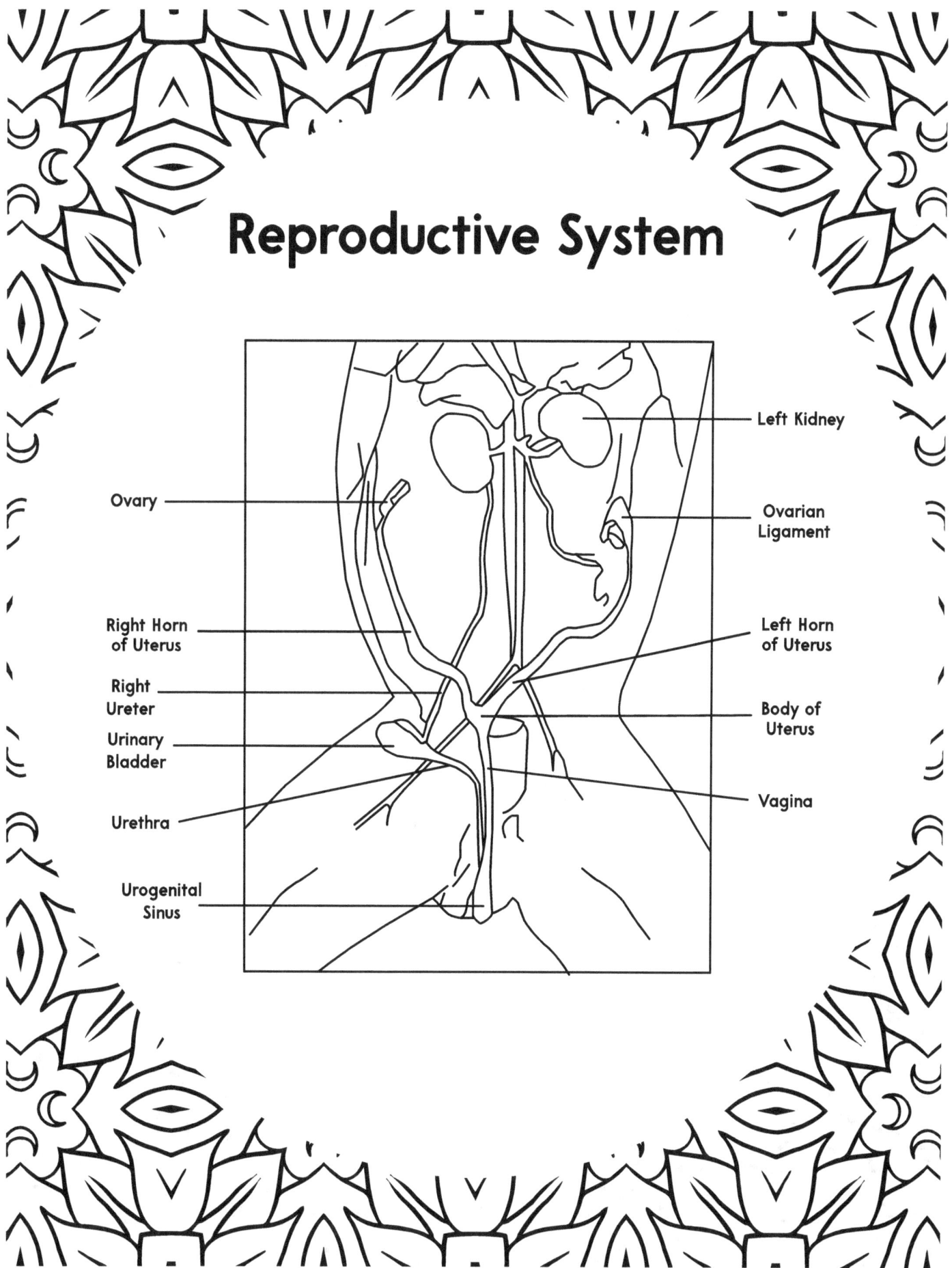

Disorders of the Pharynx in Cats

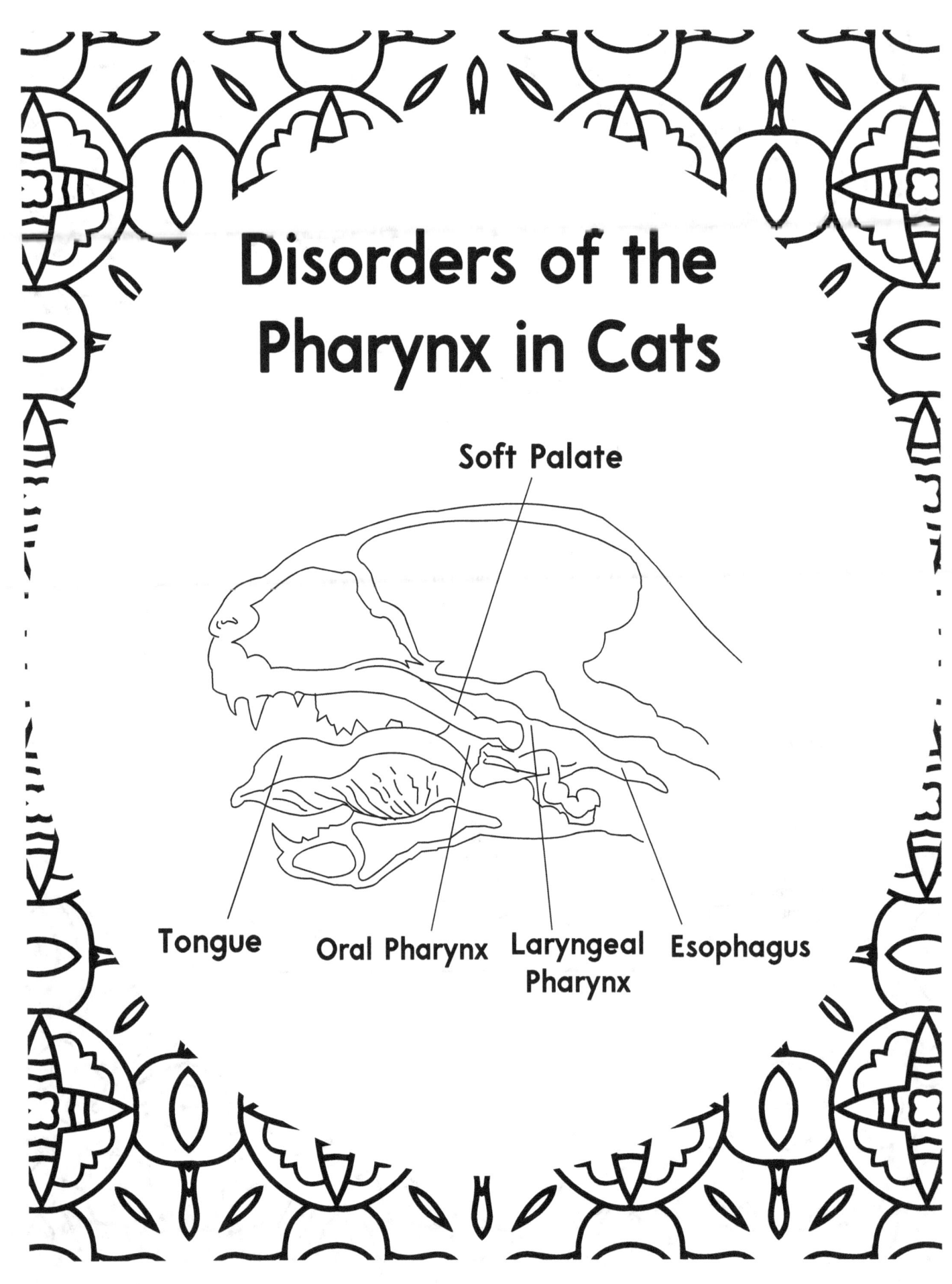

Soft Palate

Tongue   Oral Pharynx   Laryngeal Pharynx   Esophagus

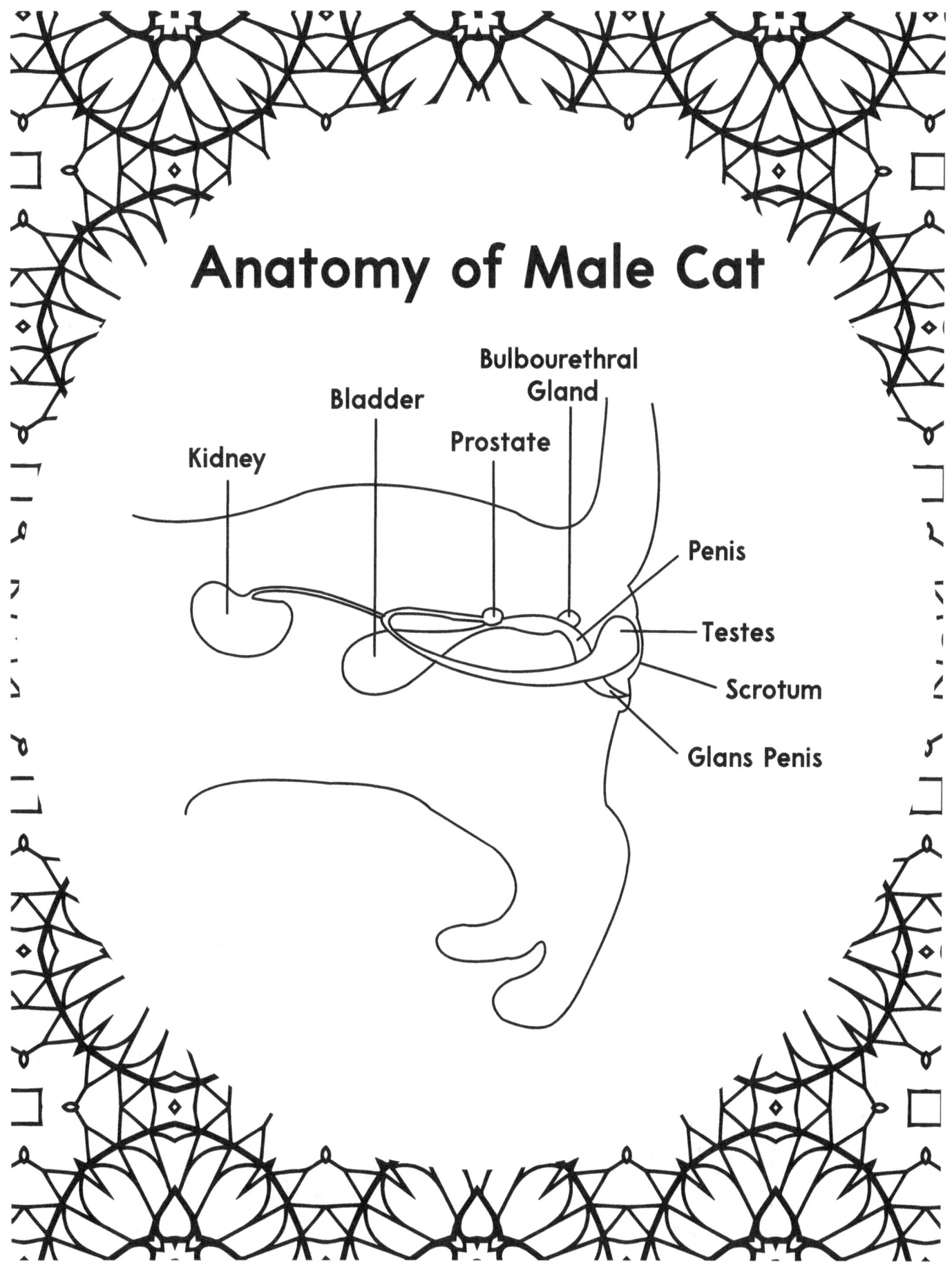

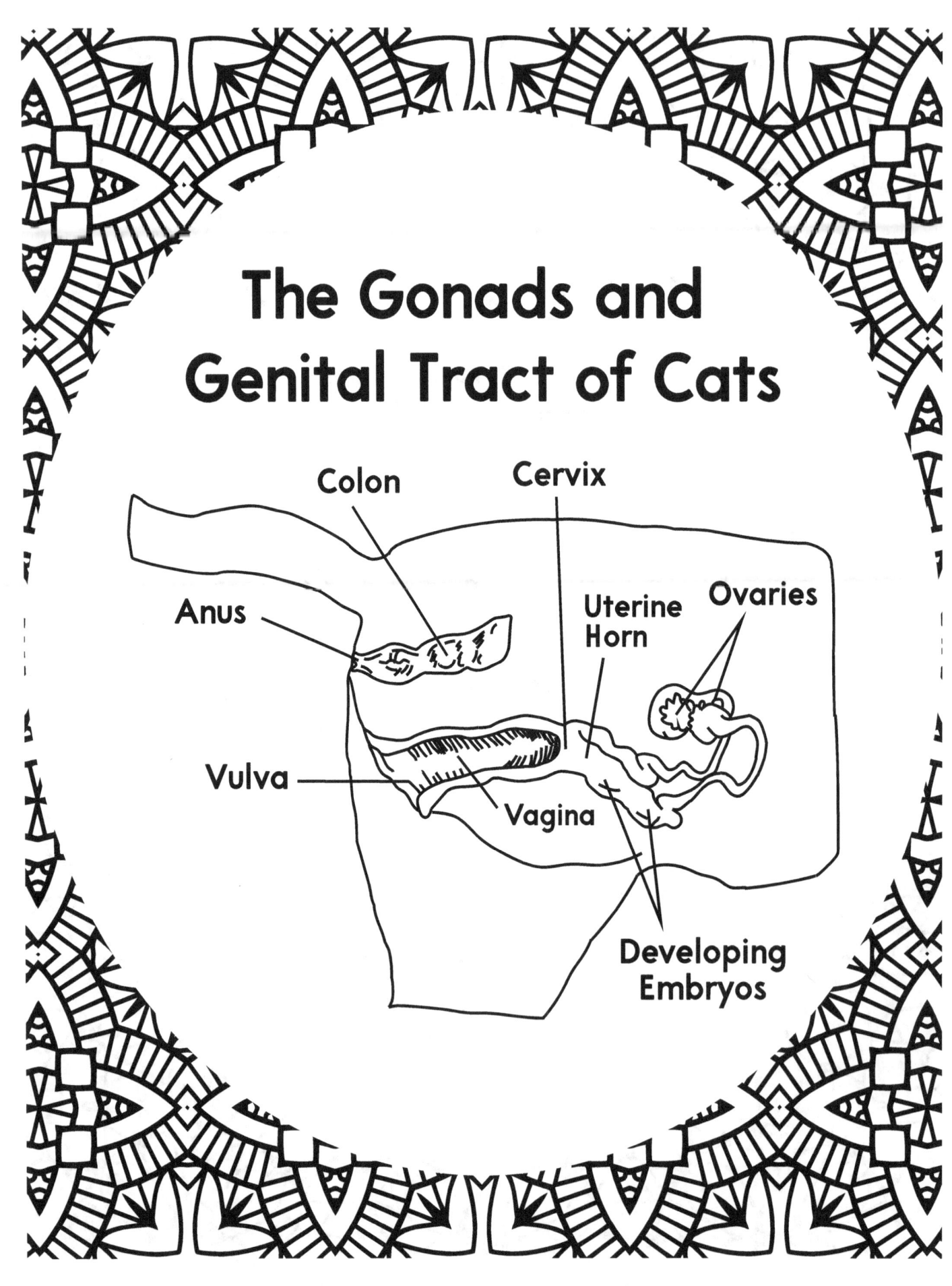

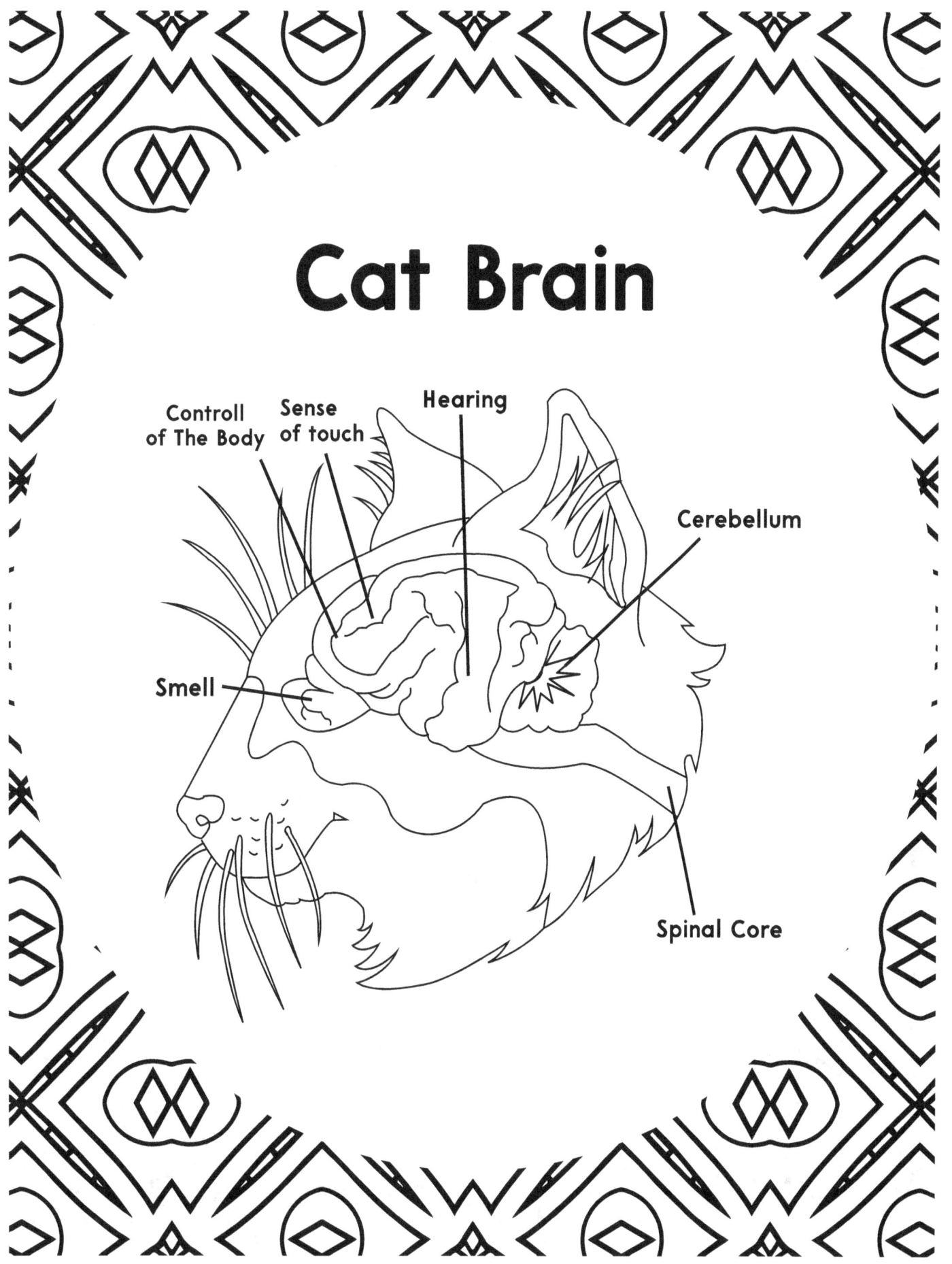

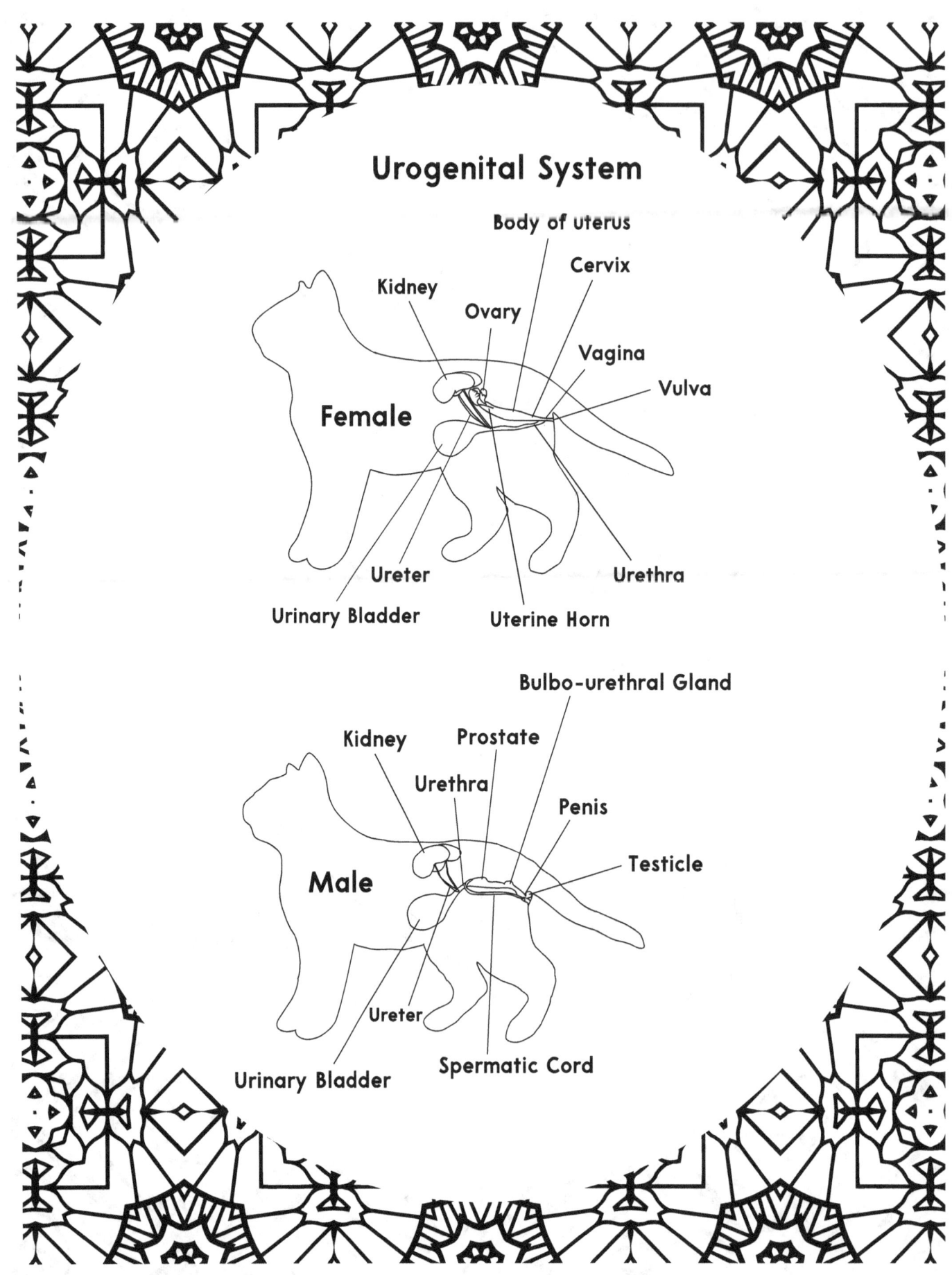

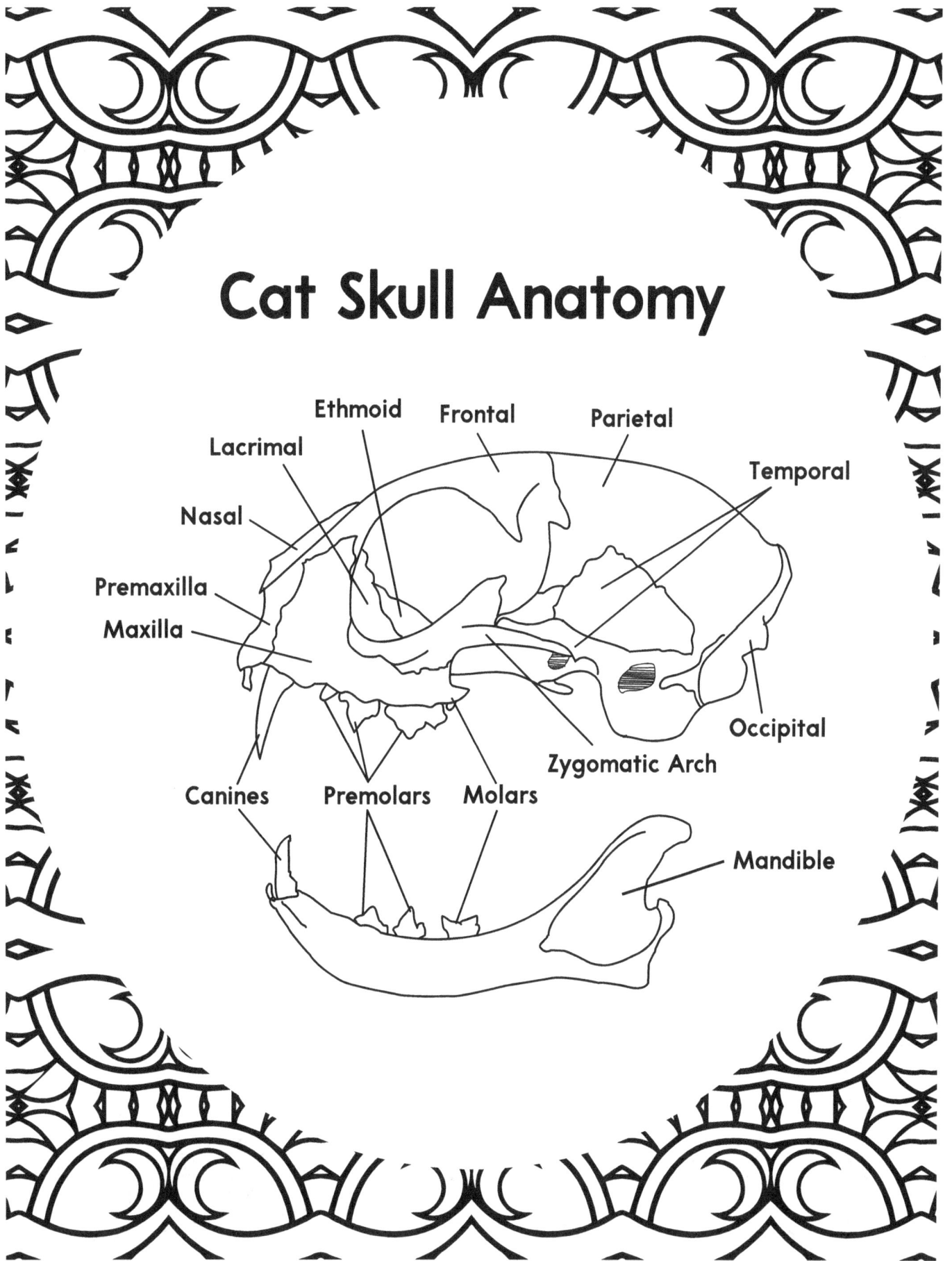

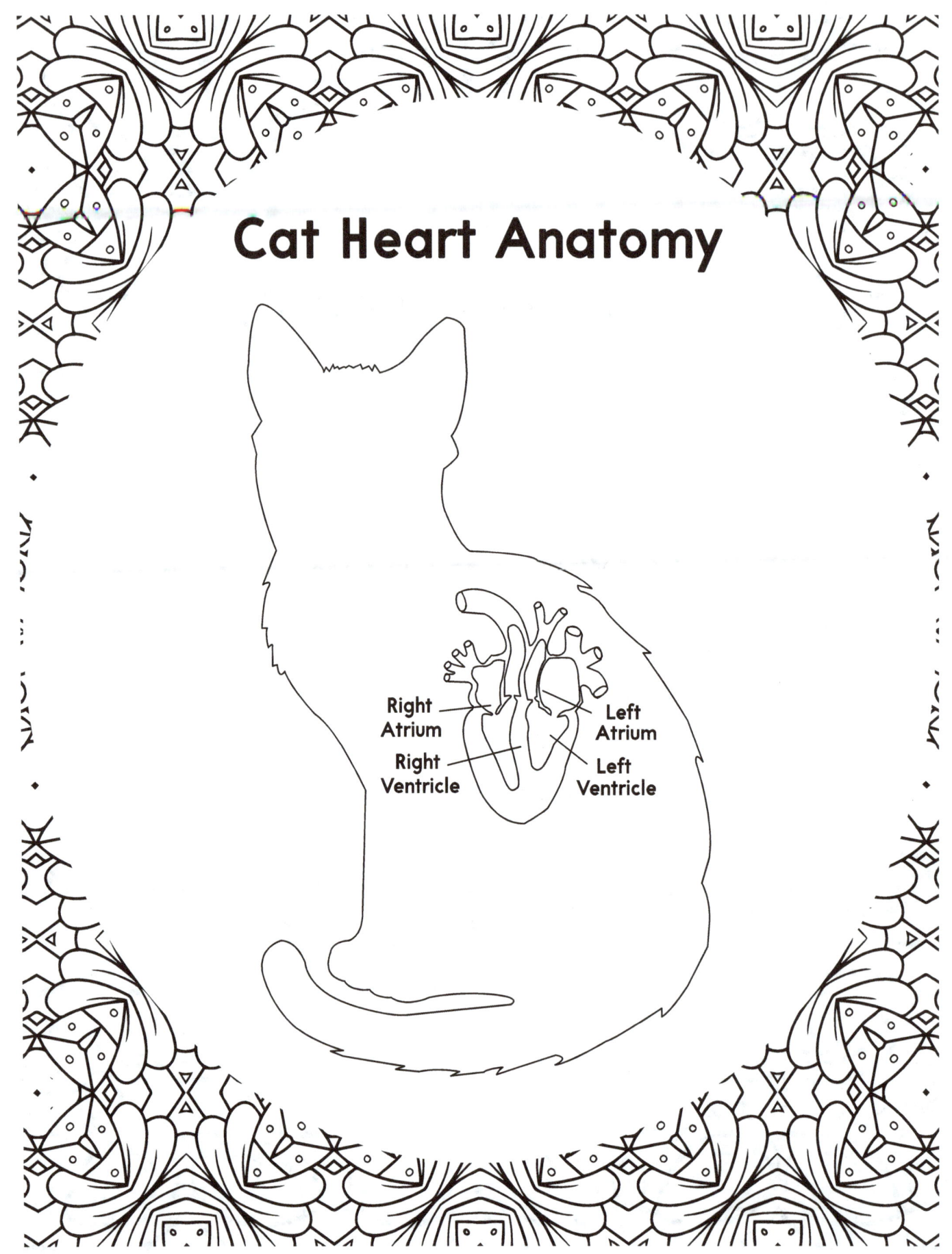

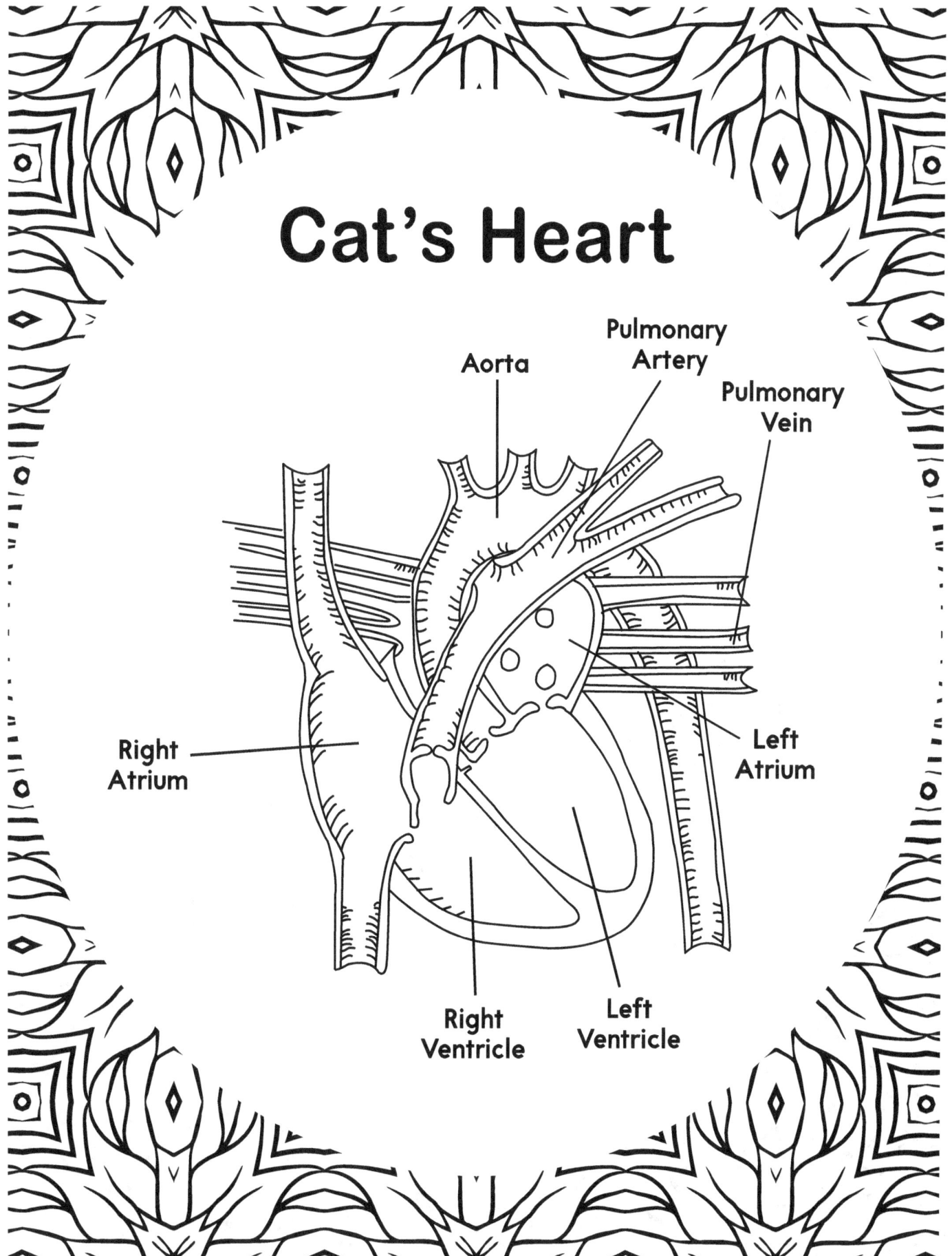

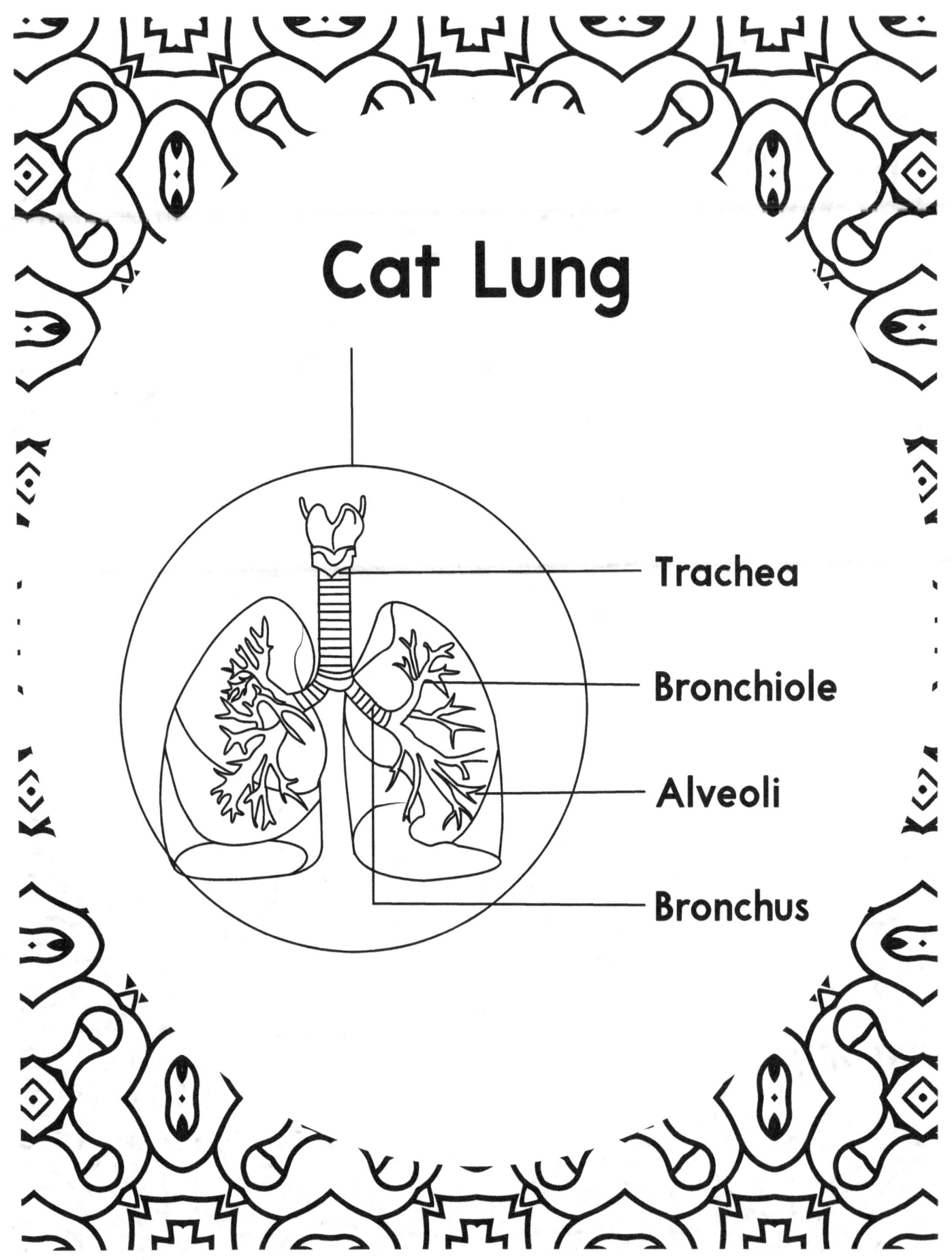

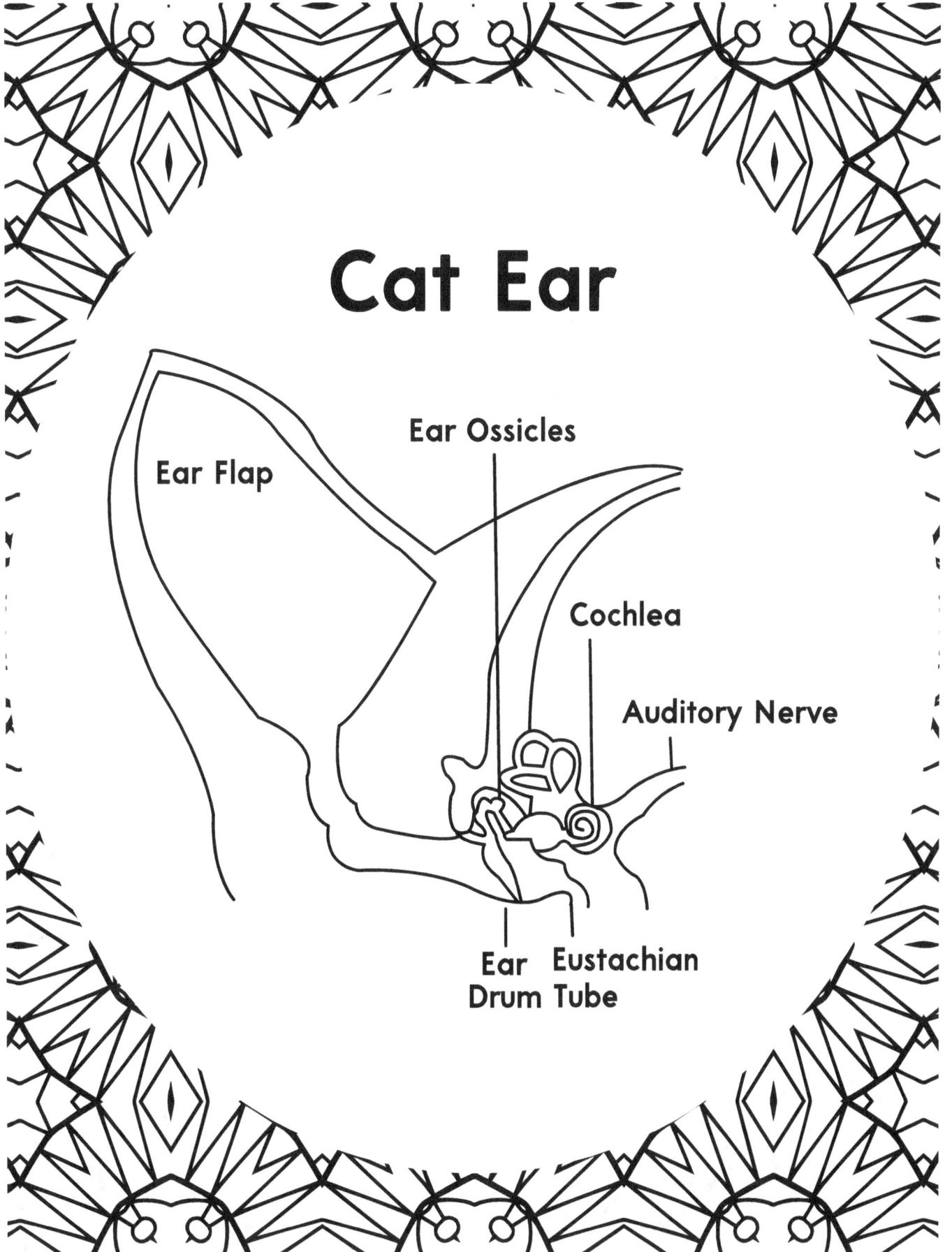

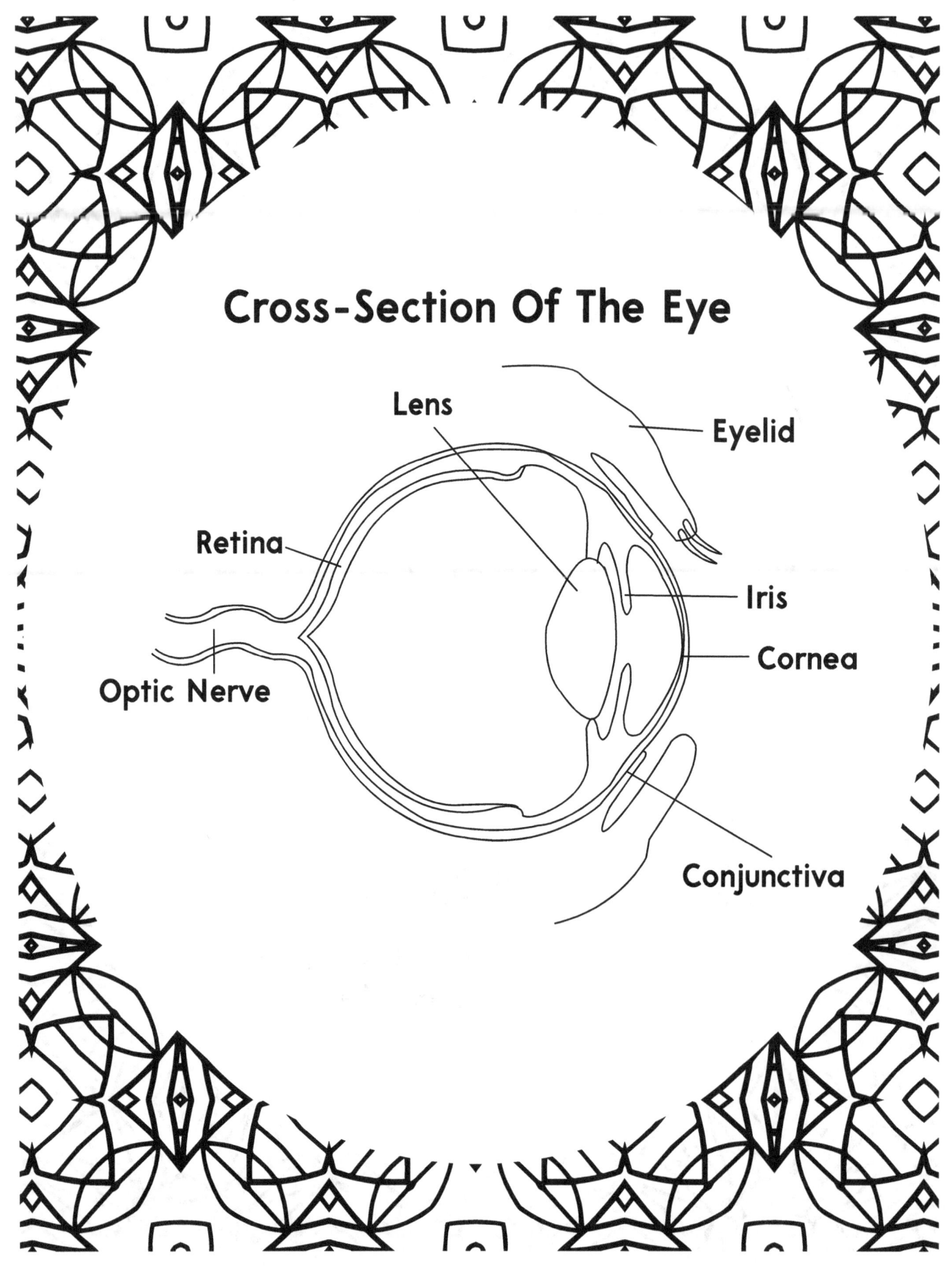

Cat's Eye

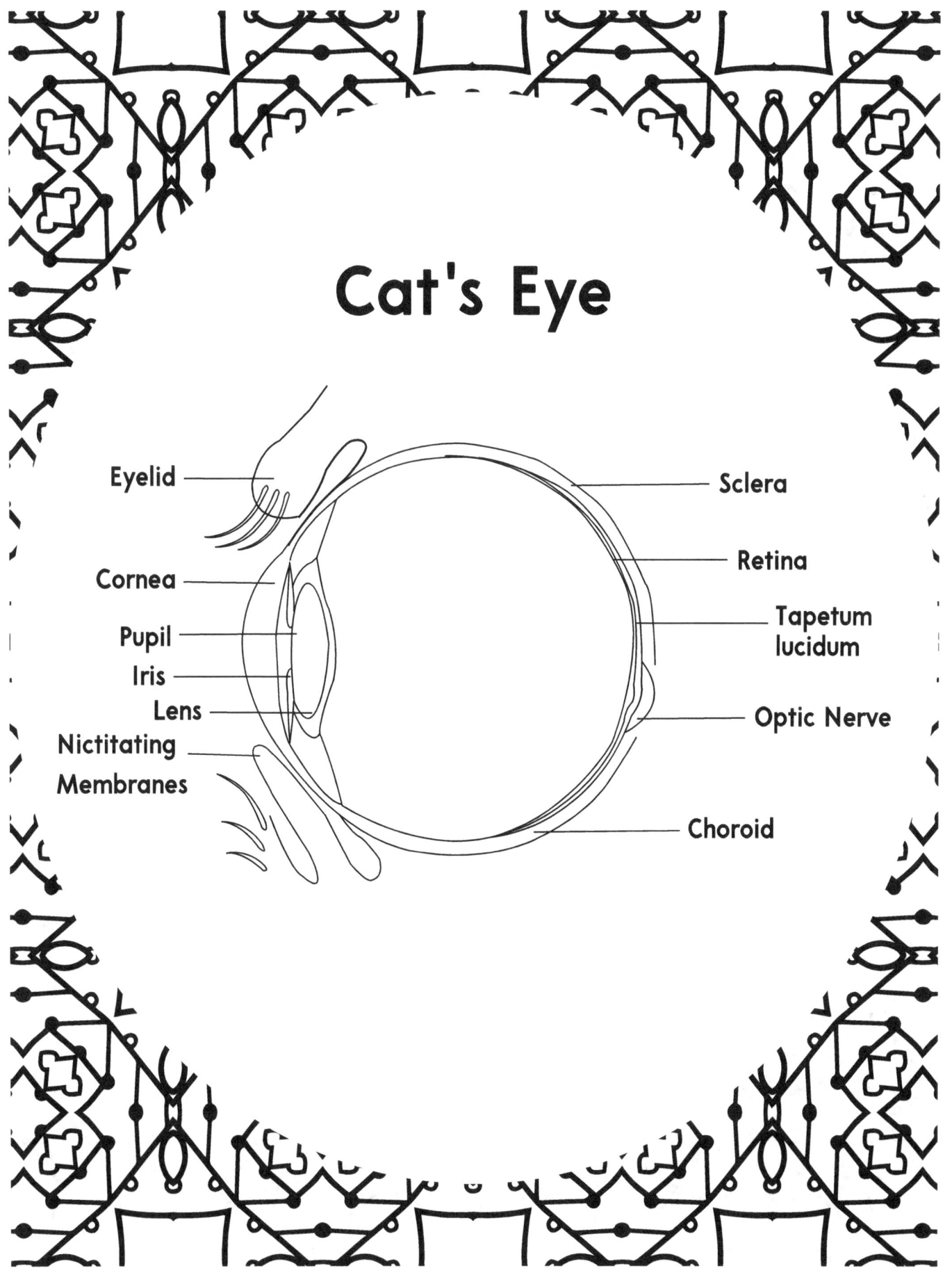

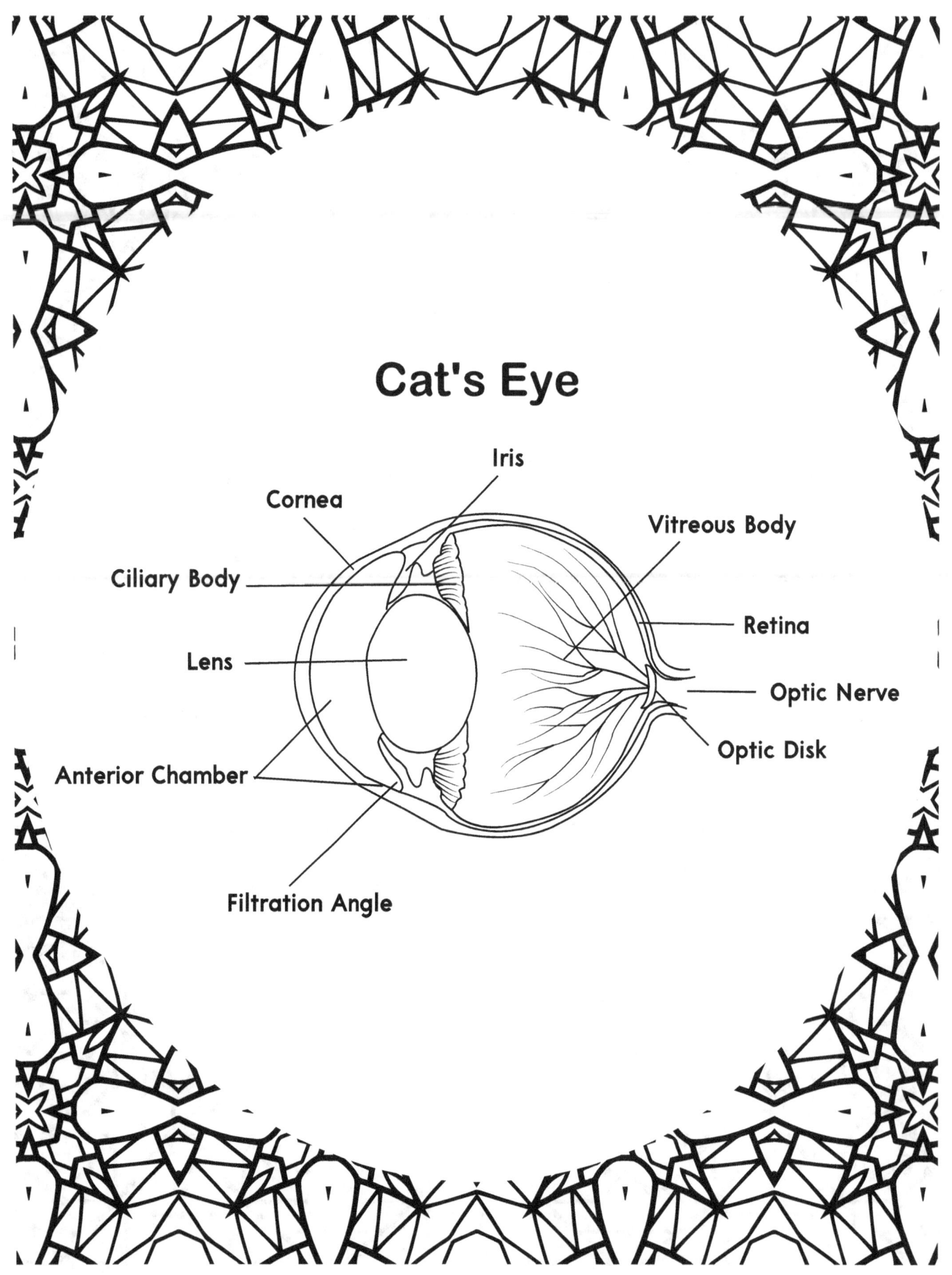

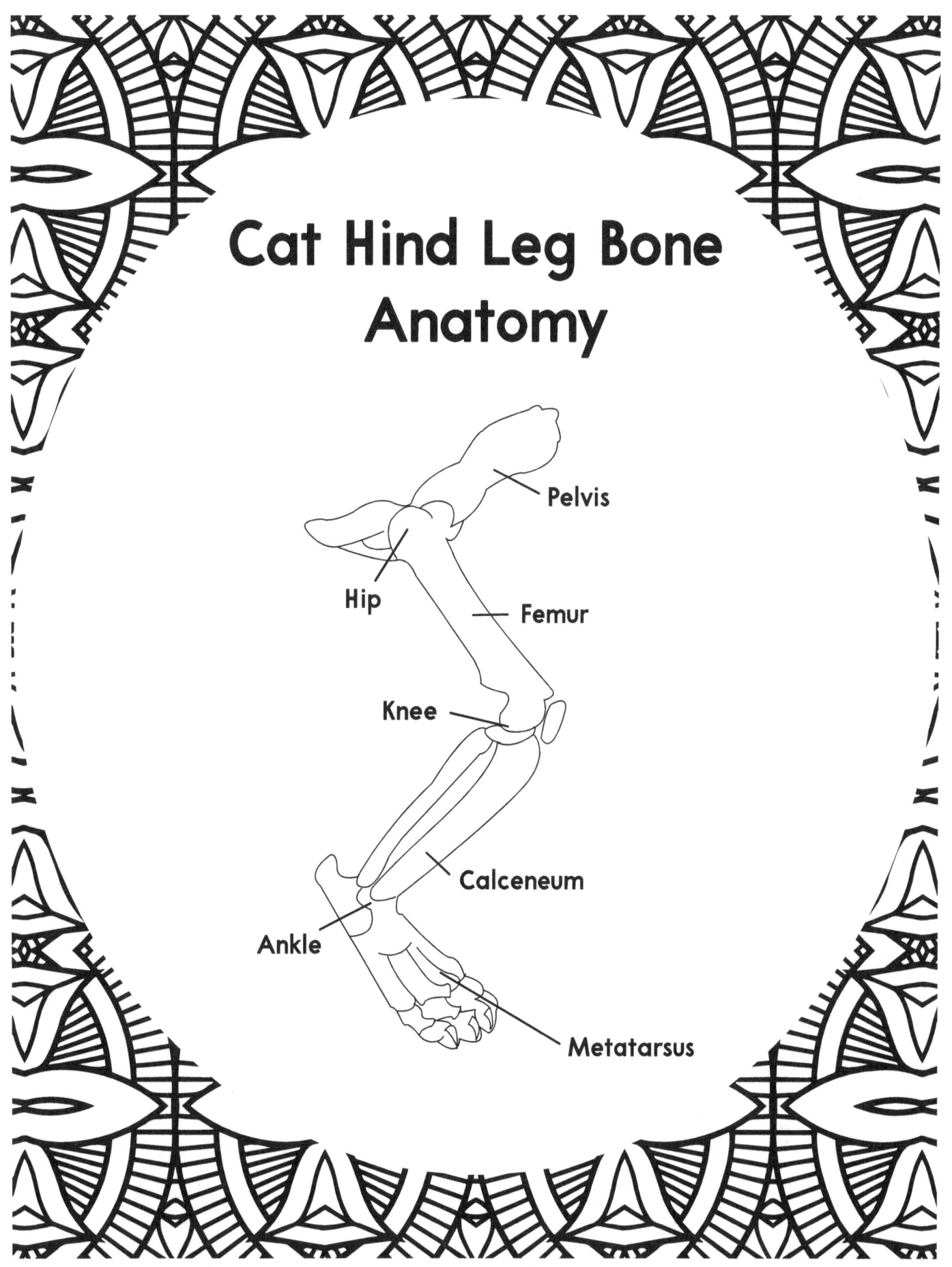

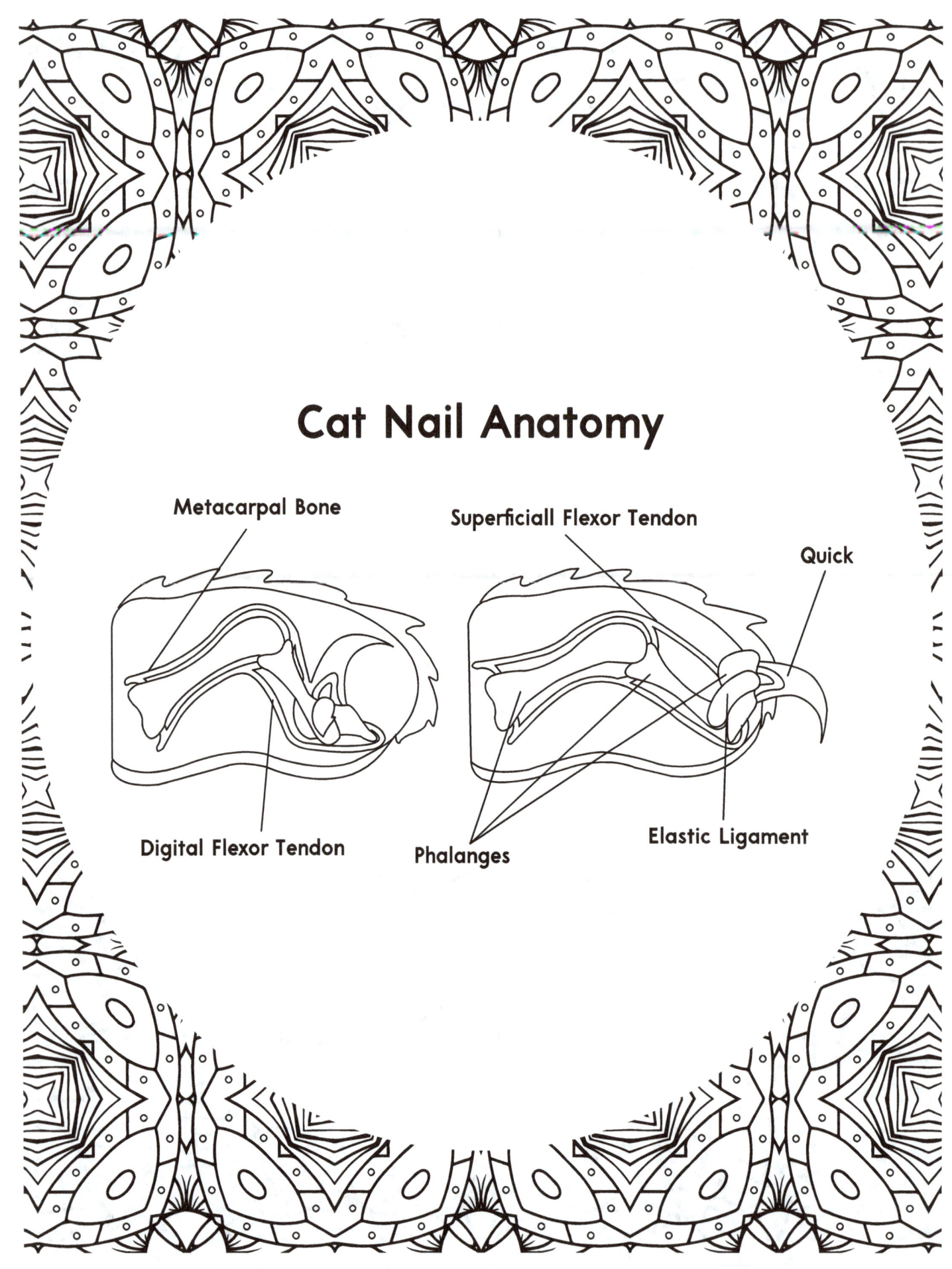

Claw of The Cat

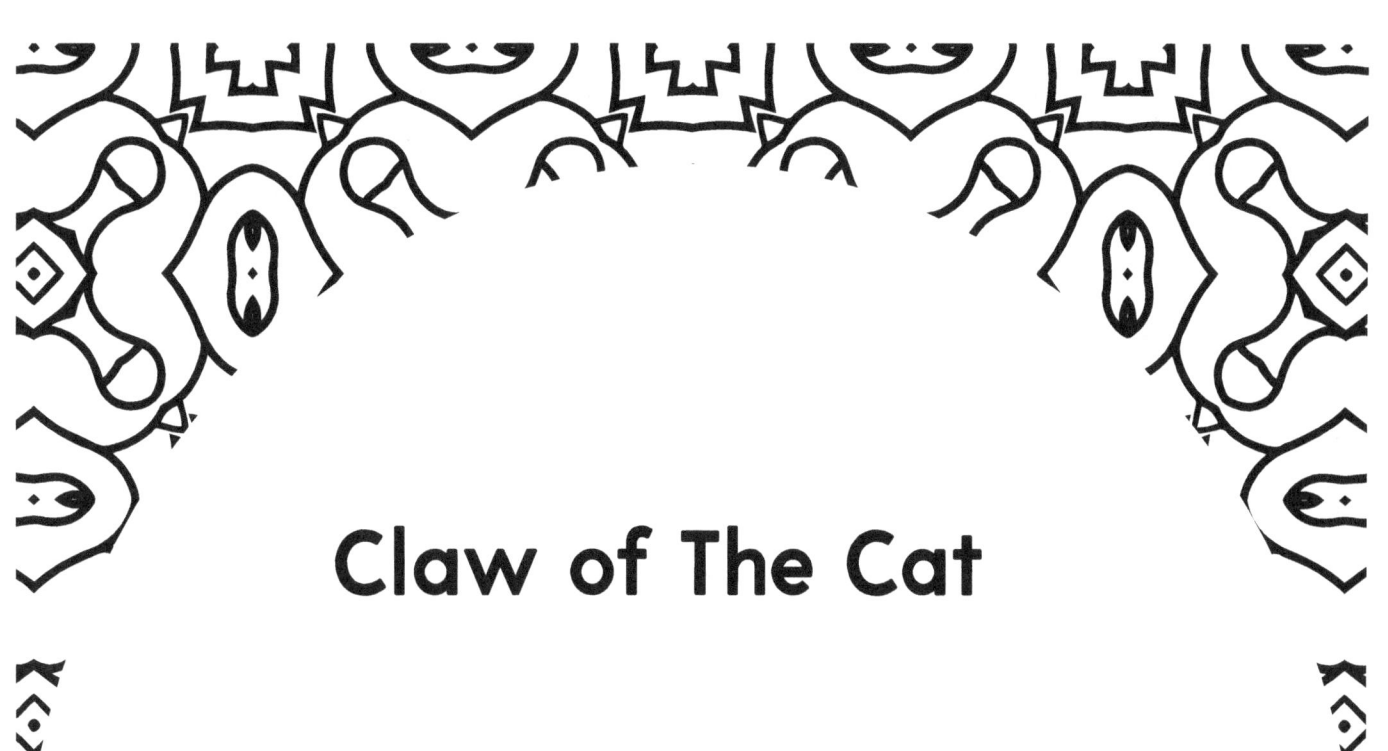

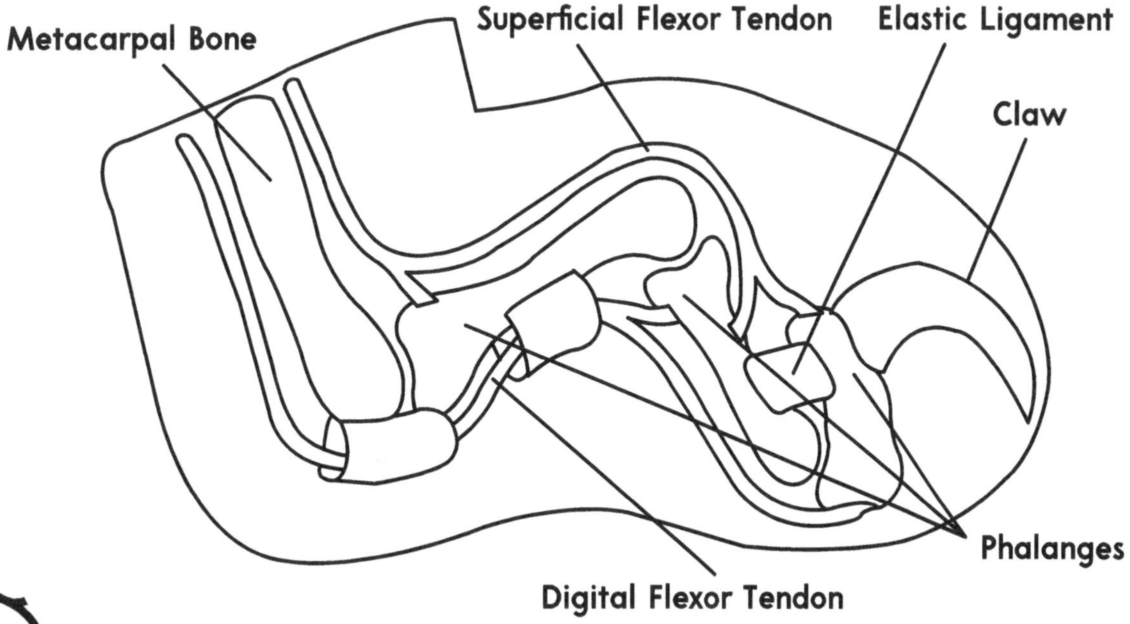

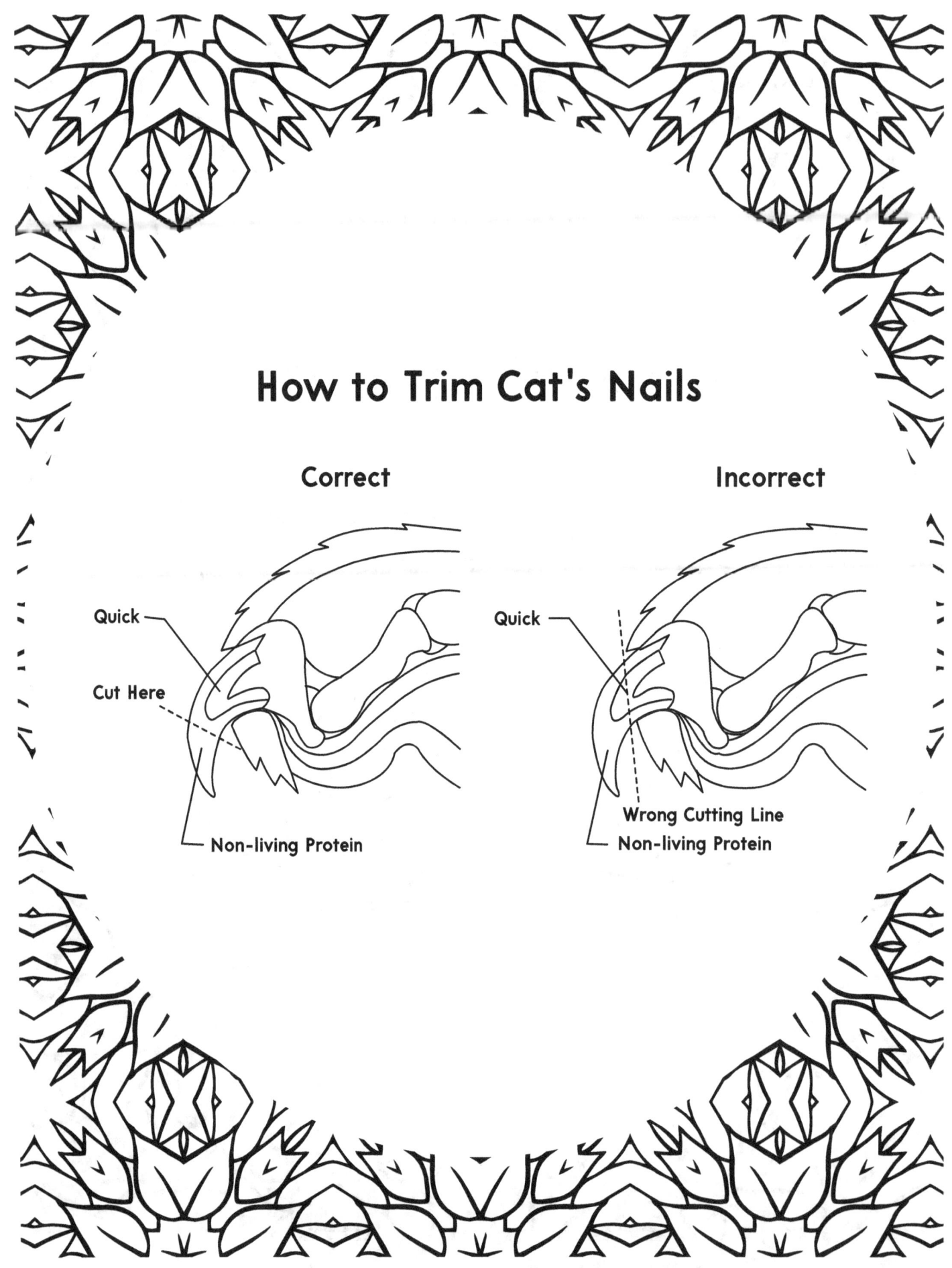

www.ingramcontent.com/pod-product-compliance
Lightning Source LLC
Chambersburg PA
CBHW080443220526
45465CB00007B/2746